Dr Alan Stewart qualified as a doctor at Guy's Hospital, London, in 1976, and spent five years specialising in hospital medicine. He became a member of the Royal College of Physicians (MRCP UK). He worked at the Royal London Homeopathic Hospital where he qualified as an MF Hom (Member of the Faculty of Homeopathy). For the last 10 years he has had a major interest in nutrition and is a founding member of the British Society for Nutritional Medicine. He is also Medical Advisor to The Women's Nutritional Advisory Service and is actively involved in educating other doctors on the subject of nutrition.

Dr Stewart co-wrote the bestselling book *Nutritional Medicine* and contributed to other books including *Beat PMT Through Diet*, *Beat Sugar Cravings*, *Inside Science*, *The Migraine Revolution* and the academic book *Post-Viral Fatigue Syndrome*. He has authored several medical papers and regularly gives lectures. Additionally, he has written articles in both the medical and popular press on various aspects of health. He has contributed to many radio programmes including the BBC *Today* programme, and has also appeared on many TV magazine shows, documentaries including BBC's *Healing Arts*, and health debates. He is also a keen gardener and a good cook.

OPTIMA

Tired all the Time

DR ALAN STEWART

An OPTIMA book

First published in Great Britain by Optima in 1993

Copyright © Alan Stewart 1993

The moral right of the author has been asserted.

A CIP catalogue record for this book is
available from the British Library.

ISBN 0 356 20763 3

Typeset in Sabon by Solidus (Bristol) Limited
Printed and bound in Great Britain by
Clays Ltd, St. Ives plc

Optima Books
A Division of
Little, Brown and Company (UK) Limited
165 Great Dover Street
London SE1 4YA

Contents

PART 2 The treatment of fatigue

Fatigue – an introduction to the problem

This is a book about fatigue and its associated conditions. It is about the problem and the solutions.

There are already a good number of books about the subject so why another one? The reason for writing this book is to try and provide a comprehensive account of the causes of fatigue and the wide number of different approaches that have brought relief to those troubled by it. Though much of the information in this book is new, much – particularly that relating to nutrition – is old, important and does not appear to be widely known.

Fatigue is a common symptom. A survey conducted in the United States found that chronic fatigue was 'a major problem' for 24 per cent of all adults attending their family doctor. A Danish study reported an even higher frequency in 1,050 forty-year-olds with 41 per cent of the women and 25 per cent of the men feeling 'tired at present'.

With such a common and sometimes persistent problem it is obvious that there is not just going to be one single cause. The evidence points overwhelmingly to there being a wide variety of causes and contributing factors of both a physical and mental nature.

This view is further supported by the findings of recent studies that report a successful outcome to trials using diverse approaches. Thus in any one individual with chronic (long-term) fatigue it seems likely that there are a number of factors at work. So if you are looking for a book with a 'magic cure' for fatigue then this is not the one for you. What this book does give is an appraisal of the causes and treatment of fatigue.

Those doctors who have specialised in the assessment and treatment of fatigue are presented with the task of determining first the actual cause(s) and then deciding on the best type of treatment(s) for their patients. Only by determining the cause can you hope to be successful in your treatment. The doctor obviously tries to be thorough but the limitations of medical resources, the limitations of his or her own knowledge and the complexities of chronic fatigue states means that he could sometimes do with a helping hand.

Often the best help comes from the patients themselves. Details about their symptoms, how their fatigue started, associated health problems, the health of other members of their family, their diet and aspects of their lifestyle are all potentially relevant.

One of the purposes of this book is to educate the patient about the relevance of these and other factors in a way that hopefully will assist the doctor, other healthcare workers and of course themselves in their recovery.

The book itself is divided into two parts. Part 1 deals with the causes of fatigue, and Part 2 deals with the treatment of fatigue. Part 1 necessarily contains a fair amount of technical detail, which I have tried to keep to a minimum whilst still being thorough. Part 2 is an easier read but some of the details about the dietary treatments are quite lengthy. The reason for this is because their success depends to a large degree on how carefully they are followed. I have also tried to anticipate the type of questions that often arise when dietary treatments are undertaken.

Part 1 also includes some case histories taken entirely from patients whom I have seen over the last thirteen years of my time in private practice, much of which has been spent specialising in nutrition. Some of the cases I have had the good fortune to help while many others have been assisted by colleagues of mine. Part 2 has hopefully been made more digestible by the inclusion of menu plans for the different diets and practical tips and guidelines about tackling the problem of chronic fatigue.

For those who are interested in the science behind the observations and recommendations made, I have included the key references in the Appendix which also contains a Glossary, a Further Reading List, a List of Useful Addresses and details of the Medical Assessment of Patients with Chronic Fatigue. I have included the latter because there is very strong evidence that between 10 and 15 per cent of patients going to their doctor to complain of chronic fatigue have a hidden physical illness or active hidden infection. This imposes a severe test for the doctor, particularly when treating those who have a fever or serious symptoms, so I have passed on some guidelines for doctors taken from certain expert texts.

I need to say a few important words about the use of the term Chronic Fatigue for diagnosis.

Throughout most of the book I have favoured the use of the term 'chronic fatigue' to describe those with fatigue which has been present for several weeks, months or longer and is of a debilitating nature. I have a strong preference for the use of the term chronic fatigue which is particularly popular in the United States and is becoming more popular elsewhere. The advantage of this term is that it is descriptively accurate without making any assumptions about the cause or the pathology (nature of the disease process) for that particular patient. Post-viral syndrome is a very useful term for describing those patients who have fatigue that followed a viral infection, and ME (myalgic encephalomyelitis) is useful for describing a group of patients with a particular group of symptoms such as headache, poor concentration and muscle pains accompanying their severe fatigue. However, we now know that there are no specific diagnostic tests for these conditions and it appears increasingly likely that in the majority of patients with fatigue there are a large number of potential causative and contributing factors. So it is less confusing to simply stick with the term chronic fatigue.

This may offend some purists but the term chronic fatigue does cover all types of fatigue states whatever their cause, pattern of symptoms or underlying pathology. Also it has been my very certain experience that too specific a label can be misleading for both the patient and the doctor.

Finally this is an optimistic book. Some of those who are reading this book may have got the impression that chronic fatigue rarely if ever improves. Certainly the media has paid undue attention to those who have been unfortunate enough to have found little to help ease their fatigued state. But the evidence from published medical papers (which has been confirmed by my own experience) is that not only do a significant number of sufferers get better by themselves but that there are numerous valid treatment approaches. Many of these approaches present the sufferer with the opportunity of doing something positive and scientifically based to help him- or herself.

That is enough for an introduction. I hope you find the book useful and exhaustive in the sense of being thorough without being exhausting.

PART 1

The causes of fatigue

1

The physical causes of fatigue

Investigating fatigue as a symptom is like opening Pandora's box. Pandora, a figure from Greek mythology, had a box which when opened released a host of ills that, as the story had it, befell mankind from that day on. Similarly the doctor who is confronted with a patient with fatigue that has been severe enough to disrupt work, home or social life also has an overwhelming number of physical ills to consider in the diagnosis and assessment of that patient's health.

It is not feasible nor desirable for everyone with fatigue to be tested for every possible physical cause. Performing all the blood tests alone would risk death of the patient by exsanguination (drainage of blood)! Like everything that is practicable in medicine there has to be a system. This brief chapter is about how that system works so that the next few chapters, some of which are technical and involved, will be more understandable.

FATIGUE – HOW SHOULD IT BE TACKLED?

First of all you should know that the medical profession takes fatigue very seriously and help is there for you to overcome it. There has been a great deal of research and there have been many medical articles written on this subject to help doctors tackle the problem. Most are excellent in the recommendations they make about assessing the individual patient with chronic fatigue. Some doctors, anticipating quite rightly that a simple treatable physical illness will only be found in a modest percentage of cases, warn against putting too much emphasis on finding an elusive physical cause. It is important to achieve a sensible balance between the need to investigate and the need to avoid expensive, time-consuming investigations that will only serve to distract the patient and doctor alike from some of the more practical ways in which the fatigue can be positively tackled using a broad-based approach.

The first duty, however, of the doctor is to determine if there is a physical illness causing or contributing to the fatigue. Physical illnesses are much better understood and many are more easily treatable than those with a psychological origin. Also no amount of psychotherapy or anti-depressants is going to be effective if there is a major untreated illness such as a tropical infection or anaemia. So the correct accepted approach to the patient with chronic fatigue is to tackle the physical side of the problems first.

The physical causes of fatigue

These can be broadly divided up into several distinct groups. There might be more than one physical factor from more than one of the categories below. Also, and most importantly, the presence of a physical illness or problem does not exclude the psychological and social aspects of illness. That said, here are the main physical factors that cause chronic fatigue:

- Following an infective illness, especially a viral one.
- A continuing infective illness.
- A hidden physical illness.
- A nutritional problem.

Most medical authorities would happily accept the first three categories but not necessarily the last. The evidence for each will be reviewed in some detail in subsequent chapters, and I will give a brief outline of each now.

It may be helpful to look first at the findings of those who have researched the physical causes of fatigue.

What the research says:

In the last twelve years, there have been at least eight medical publications reporting on how common physical illnesses have been found in patients with chronic fatigue syndrome. The findings of some of these papers are particularly relevant and interesting. The first of these was published in 1980 by Dr John D. Morrison, a family practitioner from Denver, Colorado. His review of 176 patients was particularly revealing. After very careful physical assessment, he considered that seventy-two had psychological problems only, twenty-one had psychological and physical problems combined, and sixty-nine had physical problems alone. He discovered a wide variety of both serious and minor health problems, ranging from recent viral infections, heart, lung, thyroid and liver disease, arthritis and even some with nutritional deficiencies.

A number of other studies have indicated that thyroid disease, in particular, may occur in some 4–5 per cent of patients with depression or other psychiatric illnesses. Though this is not the same as chronic fatigue syndrome, it still occurs often enough for many doctors to consider thyroid hormone problems in patients with chronic fatigue states as a matter of routine.

There are also a number of studies from Canadian and American workers who have assessed large groups of patients with chronic fatigue. As a rule, evidence of recent viral infection, especially with Epstein-Barr virus (the virus responsible for glandular fever) is a not infrequent finding. This underlines how important it is that patients with chronic fatigue syndrome are assessed carefully from both the physical as well as the psychological perspective.

A recent British study from a group at the John Radcliffe Hospital in Oxford, led by Dr Michael Sharpe, published their findings in the *British Medical Journal* in 1992. Their survey of 200 adult patients with chronic fatigue revealed that some 10 per cent had minor blood abnormalities which indicated a recent infection; an underlying blood disorder; poor immunity or mild liver problems.

There is, therefore, no substitute for doctors taking care to listen to what their patients tell them about the type of physical and other complaints that they have, to examine them thoroughly, and to perform a number of basic and if necessary specialised tests. Further details relevant to this are given in the appendix on pages 307–319.

I will now consider the four categories of physical problems causing fatigue in more detail.

Fatigue following an infective illness

This is perhaps the most familiar cause of fatigue to many people. It can almost certainly follow infection with a wide variety of viruses including glandular fever (Epstein-Barr virus) and the echoviruses that are thought by some to be responsible for many cases of myalgic encephalomyelitis (ME). Thus the terms post-viral fatigue syndrome (PVFS) or perhaps more correctly post-infective fatigue syndrome are also used.

The diagnosis is usually made when there is:

- A history of fatigue beginning at the time of, or shortly after a febrile (feverish) illness.
- A variety of physical or mental symptoms.
- No evidence for another outright cause for the fatigue.

A low level fever, up to 38.6°C (101.5°F), can be a feature of this category, but is not always present. Subtle changes in the functioning of the immune system, muscles and nerves have also been found in these patients and this probably lies behind the many different physical and mental symptoms that can occur either mildly or severely.

There is no definitive diagnostic test for the vast majority of patients in this category. There is also no clear-cut and uniformly effective treatment. Often a variety of physical, lifestyle and adaptive measures are tried by the sufferer. Fortunately there is a significant natural recovery rate in those with this diagnosis but some people experience long-standing disability.

Fatigue due to a continuing and usually treatable infection

Sometimes, albeit rarely, fatigue may be the most obvious symptom of a hidden active infection and the reason a patient consults their doctor. In post-infective fatigue syndromes, the original infection is not considered to be still active in the usual sense. Though this possibility is rare it should be considered in anyone with a continuing fever regardless of duration.

There are a wide variety of potential infecting organisms including viruses, bacteria, yeasts and small and large parasites. Many of these potential ills are confined to the tropics or sub-tropics but some are found closer to home (Europe, North America, Australia and New Zealand). Often these infections arise from close contact with animals – domestic, farm or wild – or after an insect bite which transmits the culprit germ.

There are also a number of other chronic and hidden bacterial infections that are acquired 'at home' that can also cause fatigue, fever and often but not always other symptoms. The diagnosis of an active hidden infection is suspected when:

- There is a fever especially if it is not mild.
- There are a number of either serious or specific symptoms.
- There is a history of foreign travel, contact with animals or insect bites (not always necessary).
- There are signs of a specific infection.
- Abnormal blood test results suggest that this is a possibility.

The diagnosis is made either when the actual infecting organism is isolated from the blood, sputum, faeces or urine, or there is indirect evidence of a specific type of infection usually as a result of a blood test or X-ray.

It may be difficult from the first assessment to determine the likelihood of an active hidden infection in someone with a chronic slight fever who has not been abroad because of the similarity with true post-infective fatigue syndrome. Making an accurate diagnosis is essential as virtually all of these infections are highly treatable when the appropriate antibiotics are used.

Fatigue due to a hidden physical illness

This is an important cause of fatigue, and every doctor, physician and psychiatrist should be familiar with the possible physical causes of fatigue, some of which are not easy to diagnose. The possible conditions include: arthritis, hormonal problems, cancer, side-effects of drugs, certain environmental poisons, alcohol and a wide range of other diseases affecting the heart, lungs, kidneys, bowels, liver and blood. The symptoms of such illnesses often provide a clue as to their identity. However, the picture can be misleading. For example, the presence of a fever can also be caused by one of these non-infective physical disorders. Some of these illnesses are due to common conditions appearing in an unusual manner and some are due to rare conditions; as rare as you can get. Often, but not always, a careful initial assessment will give some idea as to the likelihood of the fatigue being caused by a hidden physical illness. The diagnosis should be suspected when:

- There is significant loss of weight.
- In older patients with chronic fatigue.
- There is a prolonged illness with no improvement.
- The symptoms or signs of such illnesses exist.
- Initial blood tests show any abnormality.

The diagnosis is made when appropriate investigations confirm it. For almost all the possible hidden physical conditions there are satisfactory medical treatments and it is important that considerable care is taken so that any underlying condition is not overlooked. Doctors can be greatly aided by patients writing down a list of their symptoms or a brief history of their illness. In this way, important clues are less likely to be overlooked.

Expert advice from the US, as expressed by Dr Holmes

and colleagues from the Center for Disease Control, Atlanta, is that, 'periodic reconsideration of conditions (that could cause fatigue) should be standard practice in the long-term follow-up of these patients.' So some chronic fatigue sufferers may need a second opinion or to see two or more specialists if they have persistent or unusual symptoms.

Fatigue caused by hidden nutritional problems

This is a more contentious area and one that may be new to many people including medical practitioners. There is good evidence, though not conclusive, that nutritional deficiencies and possibly food allergies or intolerances may occasionally cause fatigue. Deficiency of essential vitamins, minerals and other nutrients do occur in both ill and 'healthy' populations in the United Kingdom as well as the US and other prosperous and developed countries. Severe deficiencies, which certainly can cause fatigue, are rare except in people with a disease but mild deficiencies of iron and B vitamins are relatively common and may cause mild fatigue and other minor symptoms.

Nutritional deficiencies should be suspected in a person when:

- There is a history of a poor diet or high alcohol intake.
- There is a history of weight loss or digestive problems.
- Other risk factors for nutritional inadequacy are present which I will talk more about in Chapter 6.
- Symptoms or signs suggestive of nutritional deficiency are present.

The diagnosis is made by testing for the nutrient in question and monitoring the response to treatment. The presence of a mild or severe deficiency does not rule out any other physical illness nor necessarily make the role of psychological and social factors less important.

There have been several successful trials of different nutritional treatments but these need to be looked at critically in order to determine their value and usefulness. There is significant potential in looking further at the role of nutritional factors in fatigue states in view of the effects of individual nutrients on immune system, muscle and nerve function, and the role that they play in metabolism and energy release.

Food allergy and intolerance have been even more contentious topics than nutritional deficiency. They doubtlessly can be involved in eczema, nettle rash – hives or urticaria – asthma, bowel problems, migraine headaches, some types of arthritis and a variety of other conditions. An observation of many workers in this field is that sometimes fatigue, especially when it co-exists with one of the conditions above, improves if one or more foods are excluded from the diet. There is also some laboratory evidence to support the notion that true food allergy is associated with fatigue. But diagnosis is difficult as there are few reliable blood tests for food allergy or intolerance.

The diagnosis of food allergy or intolerance should be suspected when:

- Fatigue co-exists with any of the above conditions.
- The individual is known to have pre-existing food allergies or intolerances.
- Other physical causes of fatigue have been excluded.

The diagnosis is made when blood tests clearly indicate an allergic state (this is rarely the case), and when there is significant improvement if one or more foods are avoided followed by a consistent deterioration when a particular food or foods are introduced back into the diet.

Making a diagnosis of food allergy or intolerance is often not easy and requires a certain amount of skill on the part of the doctor and considerable determination on the part of the patient. If you do discover you are allergic to a particular food or drink, managing to avoid it at all times can result in sustained benefit, but more of this later.

Unknown physical causes

Sometimes, despite the most thorough assessment, a physical cause is suspected but none is found. This creates a difficult and frustrating situation for doctor and patient alike. Doctors' statements such as, 'There is nothing physically wrong with you, so it must be in your mind', are unhelpful and anyway may be untrue. A truer and more useful statement is, 'I can find no serious physical illness at present, and therefore we have to look at what broad constructive measures can be undertaken to improve your overall health.' It is just good practice for doctors – physicians and psychiatrists alike – to be aware of the possibility that a physical illness may manifest itself later on. Occasionally, fatigue is the symptom that prompts a patient to go to the doctor and may be the only sign of an illness which does not show on initial investigations.

Most of the remainder of Part 1 of the book deals with these physical causes of fatigue. The next chapter, however, is about the relationship between chronic fatigue and mental problems as this too is an important area.

2

The mental causes of fatigue

Until recently many doctors and research workers argued that patients with chronic fatigue either have a physical illness or a psychological illness. Taking this 'either/or' approach is limiting our thinking. Just as in life generally, it is rare in medicine and nature that there is a completely black or white picture. Shades of grey are the norm. Assuming that there is a physical cause pays dividends if this is the only problem – which is true of perhaps 10 to 20 per cent of cases. Psychological factors are more common than this and may be influenced by many subtle factors both psychological and physical. If no physical cause is found then the doctor is often tempted to say to the patient that it is 'all in your mind' and leave the patient with an unacceptable diagnosis and no constructive way out.

A more useful attitude is to consider that there are usually both physical and psychological factors in all cases. Usually physical factors are addressed first but while investigations and assessment of physical health are underway it is perfectly appropriate to look at the psychological aspects of the illness.

I would like to give a brief outline of the psychological factors that may be relevant in chronic fatigue syndrome. A lot of research has been conducted in this area which I will deal with briefly.

Psychological illness as a factor in fatigue

One of the most persuasive arguments that psychological factors are relevant in chronic fatigue syndrome is that people with chronic fatigue are more likely to have a history of psychological problems than the general population before the onset of their fatigue. Furthermore, many of the mental symptoms of chronic fatigue are similar to those of depression, with some element of anxiety. There are, however, various pitfalls and limitations to these arguments.

For instance, Drs Wessely and Powell from the Institute of Psychiatry in London found that 72 per cent of a group of chronically fatigued patients had associated mental symptoms of depression or anxiety.

Dr Wood and colleagues from Liverpool found that 41 per cent of chronically fatigued patients could actually be diagnosed as psychiatric cases which is approximately two to three times the expected number of cases when compared with patients suffering from other nerve or muscle diseases or the normal population. These findings were supported by an American study on twenty-eight chronically fatigued patients by Dr M.J.P. Kruesi. However, Dr Ian Hickie and co-workers from Australia found that psychiatric problems in patients with fatigue were no more common than in the rest of the population. The differences in these findings can perhaps be explained by the fact that different populations are being examined, and that different methods of assessment are being used.

Psychological illness that existed before the onset of fatigue could, in some of the patients studied, have been caused by physical illness or poor nutritional state, which may not have been detected at first.

The assessment of depression by some psychiatrists and some psychiatric assessment questionnaires involves asking for various physical symptoms that are said to be suggestive of a depressed state. These include poor appetite, changes in sleeping habits, bowel symptoms, changes in libido and headaches. All of these symptoms have several physical causes as well as depression. Actual chronic physical ills, food intolerances, hormonal imbalances and nutritional problems can all produce a mixture of physical and psychological complaints. Also there is substantial evidence from psychiatric research that between 10 per cent and 40 per cent of psychiatric patients admitted to hospital do have a hidden physical illness which is either the sole cause of or a contributing factor to their mental state. Patients with chronic fatigue who feel depressed and may be diagnosed as suffering primarily from 'depression' should not be denied a careful and thorough physical assessment.

The association between previous psychiatric and mental problems in chronic fatigue syndrome cannot be ignored. It is probably fair to conclude that patients who go to their doctor with chronic fatigue syndrome are more likely to have experienced psychological or mental problems at some time prior to the onset of their illness.

Psychological reactions to acute infections

It has long been recognised that an acute infection can produce psychological symptoms, such as depression, either during the course of the illness or following on from it. There are many ways in which this could occur. The infection may:

- Affect the nervous system directly, causing a subtle change in its chemistry.
- Increase the demand for certain nutrients, including folic acid and vitamin C, which in turn may influence mood.
- Induce a level of physical inactivity which the sufferer is unused to and which in turn may have a depressing effect.
- Cause a suppression of appetite, weight loss and thus increased feelings of ill health.
- Cause social isolation, loss of contact with friends and workmates, and loss of self-esteem if there is a period of prolonged ill health and time off work.

In other words, you don't have to be mad to feel sad when you're ill!

Some of the best research demonstrating this has been in relation to glandular fever – infectious mononucleosis – which is caused by the Epstein-Barr virus. As long ago as 1976, Professor Peter Storey, when working at St George's Hospital, London, followed up 36 patients who had had clear-cut infectious glandular fever. One year later, five of the 20 women considered that they had moderate or severe depression or fear/anxiety problems following their illness, whereas only one had experienced such problems before the infection. Men seem much less affected than women.

A more recent study led by Dr Paul White, Senior Lecturer at St Bartholomew's Hospital, London, supported these findings. Together with general practitioners, psychologists and infectious disease specialists, a group of 249 patients recovering from a variety of infections, including glandular fever, were studied.

Their conclusions were that: a genuine fatigue syndrome exists after acute respiratory tract infections, 10 per cent of patients still had fatigue syndrome six months after glandular fever, and fatigue syndrome was different from pure depressive illness and anxiety. They also concluded that there are 'predisposing', 'precipitating' and 'perpetuating' factors of a physical and psychological nature which led Dr White and his colleagues to advocate quite rightly an holistic approach as being the best way forward.

Predisposing factors   These could include anything that influences the immune system which will include nutrition, genetic factors and psychological factors.

Precipitating factors   These include life changes, such as moving house, loss of employment, a divorce or separation as well as physical stresses, such as an operation or a viral infection.

Perpetuating factors   These may include the level of previous physical fitness, the degree of family and social support, the quality of medical advice received, the personal desire to return to work, and any underlying physical or nutritional factors that might hinder either immune function or energy levels, together with changes in immune, nerve and muscle function as a result of the viral infection itself.

Depression as a symptom of a physical illness

On a final note, it should be remembered that all fatigued patients with depression should be assessed very thoroughly for physical and nutritional factors.

3

Fatigue, viral infection and myalgic encephalomyelitis (ME)

Over the last forty or more years there have been many reports of groups of patients troubled by chronic fatigue who had evidence of a recent infection with a virus or unidentified organism. Often, but not always, these reports would describe an outbreak of an illness which caused a fever, fatigue and muscular aches and pains as the key components. Such a pattern of illness fully justified the use of the terms post-viral syndrome or myalgic encephalo-myelitis.

A number of viruses were suspected or identified both in these outbreaks and in a number of individual cases. There have been several viruses identified including that respons-ible for glandular fever, the Epstein-Barr virus.

Accordingly, many research workers around the world have found themselves with a group of patients with chronic fatigue and the following symptoms:

- A history of a viral infection.
- Continuing ill-health.
- A low-grade fever which may come and go.
- An intermittent or chronic mild sore throat.
- Painful and swollen neck glands.
- Headaches and muscular pains.
- Poor concentration and memory.
- Depression and sleep disturbance.
- Unusual sensations such as numbness or tingling.
- A variety of other physical and mental symptoms.

Although doctors doubted that there were any physical causes involved in the illness at first, this has in the last decade given way to an understanding of some of the subtle physical abnormalities that can be found. In this way we have been better able to understand why some people experience the symptoms they do.

WHAT LIES BEHIND CHRONIC FATIGUE AND ME

There is now very good evidence that those with chronic fatigue syndrome, or myalgic encephalomyelitis, can have one or more of a variety of mild physical abnormalities, which include:

- A continuing viral infection.
- A past viral infection.
- Altered function of the immune system.
- A change in muscle function.
- A change in nervous system function.

Sometimes these discoveries have been heralded as 'breakthroughs' but unfortunately so far they have not led to an effective treatment. Furthermore, none of the abnormalities described have been found in all who suffer with chronic fatigue or ME – only in a proportion of them. So we do not therefore have such a thing as 'a test for ME'.

Clearly, however, there is evidence that something, in some subtle way, has 'gone wrong'. How we put that right remains to be seen.

Evidence of chronic viral infection

Viruses are extremely small infective organisms that invade the cells of a host, be it a person, animal or plant. They are on the whole much smaller than bacteria and exist in many forms. The essential part of the virus is that it contains a piece of nuclear material which functions as a primitive brain. This contains a blueprint with information on how to replicate itself using the nutrients and chemicals available in the target or host cell. Thus a cell infected with one viral particle will eventually be overwhelmed and die, as tens or hundreds of new viral particles are made from its contents. As the infected cells die they release a variety of chemicals which stimulate the white cells of our immune system to attack the virus and produce antibodies against it. The body tries to kill the virus and limit its spread. In the ensuing battle many cells die including some of those of the immune system itself, as well as those infected by the virus. The release of even more chemicals is often associated with general feelings of ill health as well as local evidence of inflammation, such as the pain and swelling you experience with a sore throat or swollen infected neck glands.

There are thousands of viruses, just as there are many bacteria, and they have different characteristics. Most of those that are relevant to this section enter the body via the mucus membranes of the nose, mouth, throat and lungs, or through the gastro-intestinal tract. They spread through the body via the bloodstream. Some have developed an ability to hide inside muscle cells, cells of the nervous system or even in white cells of the blood. By so doing they escape some of the attacks of the immune system itself. Some ingenious germs also produce their own chemicals that paralyse or suppress the immune system in order to increase their own chances of survival. So, as you can imagine, there is often a battle royal which sometimes develops into a slow and prolonged contest rather like guerilla warfare.

Modern diagnostic techniques over the last twenty years have been able to identify the presence of hidden viral particles in some patients with chronic fatigue. One of the best known of these chronic hidden viruses is the Epstein-Barr virus. It is the commonest cause of glandular fever (or infectious mononucleosis). Quite often the infection is silent or mild, only causing a sore throat for a few days. The vast majority of patients recover within a week or two after having the sore throat and glandular enlargement but a few go on to develop a chronic illness. Sophisticated tests for the glandular fever virus have become available recently, and these may be useful in detecting those who have a chronic infection or episodes when the virus is reactivated, which is now known to occur in some susceptible adults and children.

There is good evidence that active E-B virus infection occurs in patients with persistent unexplained fatigue, both from the United States and the United Kingdom. Professor T.J. Hamblin from the Department of Haematology at the Royal Victoria Hospital, Bournemouth in the United Kingdom, showed in 1983 that some patients with chronic ill health after glandular fever had minor changes in the immune system. Other researchers have suggested that some patients with chronic symptoms following E-B virus infection do not produce a response to the virus which is

CCC

adequate to kill it. Consequently, the E-B virus infection passes into a chronic phase and may reactivate from time to time. Research work suggests that this may be the case in up to 20 per cent of patients with chronic fatigue syndrome or ME.

Case History

Lisa Pope

Lisa was a fourteen-year-old schoolgirl who eighteen months previously had had a proven infection with Epstein-Barr virus which produced fever, sore throat, greatly enlarged neck glands and significant fatigue. She had several weeks off from school, but made a satisfactory recovery until symptoms recurred fifteen months later. It seemed that she had true chronic Epstein-Barr virus infection.

Blood tests had shown that she was not anaemic or iron deficient. Serum zinc, however, was modestly reduced at 10.4 micromols per litre (the normal range being 11.5–20).

I encouraged her to take supplements of zinc, multivitamins, and eat a high protein diet. After six weeks, both she and her mother had noticed a considerable improvement in her energy levels, she felt less depressed and was able to work better in the evenings. Her disturbed sleeping pattern also seemed to be a little improved.

The changes that she had made in her diet were relatively simple. Ensuring a good intake of protein will naturally increase the intake of zinc, and I suggested that she tail off all her supplements after three months.

Her improvement could easily have been spontaneous

but it seemed only common sense to recommend a nutritious diet and a brief course of supplements to correct a mild deficiency and perhaps enhance the rate of natural recovery.

The Epstein-Barr virus is one of a family of viruses known as the herpes viruses. Other members of this group include herpes simplex (responsible for cold sores and genital herpes), herpes zoster (responsible for shingles) and cytomegalovirus which causes a glandular fever-like illness. They and other herpes viruses may all cause chronic or recurrent infections with their own particular pattern of symptoms.

In Scotland, Professor Behan, Professor of Neurology at the University of Glasgow, has been at the forefront of research into patients with post-viral fatigue syndrome. He and co-workers had initially found that many patients with post-viral syndrome had evidence of infection with another virus called Coxsackie B.

Their most recent work suggests that this was simply a reflection of a community infection with this virus, which causes a mild fever, sore throat or cold. Again, Coxsackie B is but one of several of many enteroviruses (viruses that cause gastro-enteritis and 'flu'). They are common infectious agents which gain access to the body, again via mucus membranes. Polio virus is yet another one of the enteroviruses. It has been estimated that everyone is exposed to about one enterovirus a year, usually in the summer months. A small proportion of those infected may go on to develop symptoms of chronic fatigue or ME.

Professor James Mowbray, Professor of Immunopathology at St Mary's Hospital Medical School, London, has also been involved in extensive research into the role of enteroviruses in ME. In 1988, he and colleagues published in the *Lancet* medical journal evidence that a larger than normal percentage of patients with post-viral fatigue syndrome had an antibody directed against an enterovirus particle termed VP-1. Thus, some patients with chronic post-viral fatigue syndrome seemed to be fighting a hidden infection with an enterovirus. This seemed to be the pattern in some 50 per cent of the patients they investigated. Another group of researchers from the National Hospital for Nervous Diseases in London, have made similar findings in their group of patients with ME. This time finding that some 30 per cent of cases were positive for VP-1, compared with 12 per cent of non-sufferers.

In conclusion, the evidence suggests that something like 30 to 50 per cent of patients with chronic fatigue are responding to a chronic viral infection. It is quite possible that other hidden viruses, yet to be identified, may also be found more frequently in patients with chronic fatigue syndrome or ME than in the normal healthy population. What then needs to be determined is why some people seem to be especially susceptible to the long-term adverse health effects of a viral infection and what can be done about it. Suggestions as to the types of treatments that are currently available and can be effective can be found in Part 2 of the book.

Evidence of altered function of the immune system

Viruses can also affect the immune system. As already mentioned, instead of being attacked by white cells and antibodies (proteins that are designed to stick to and destroy the virus) the virus can actually alter the immune system in a way that allows it to survive. An 'intelligent' virus can thus try to suppress the immune system, which then allows the virus to survive in a chronic form. The results of studies of immune function in patients with chronic fatigue syndrome are extremely complicated. For the technically minded, the main findings include: 'Decreased function of natural killer cells and macrophages, reduced mitogenic response of lymphocytes, B-subset changes and activation of CD8 cells.'

In more simple terms the immune system is either not functioning efficiently or is being kept busy as a result of a chronic infection.

A group of American workers, Drs Landay, Jessop, Lennette and Levy from various centres in the United States, have found in a study of 147 individuals with chronic fatigue syndrome that many of them have evidence of increased immune activity. Certain cells in the immune system that reduce excessive immune activity are themselves reduced. In other words, the handbrake has been taken off some of the immune system in some patients. They did not find any association between this particular immune abnormality and any specific virus infection in this group of patients. Like others, they observed that in some patients these abnormalities persisted for a year or more, and that in those who improved, their improvement was accompanied by a return to normal in some of the immunological abnormalities.

It should be mentioned, for the sake of completeness, that there are some well-known and more serious immune abnormalities that may occasionally occur in a few patients with chronic fatigue syndrome. Reduced levels of specialised proteins – immunoglobulins A and G – that are directed against infecting organisms, including bacteria and viruses, do occur in a small percentage of the normal population and in some people with chronic fatigue.

Evidence of a change in muscle function

There is additionally good evidence that there are subtle changes in the muscles of some patients with chronic fatigue syndrome. Firstly, it should be pointed out that immobility, for any reason, results in muscle wasting and changes in the cell structure of the muscles. Nutritional deficiencies, underlying physical illness and muscle diseases can all cause loss of muscle bulk and muscle weakness. Reduction in muscle size, however, is rarely found in patients with chronic fatigue, except when it is due to lack of use.

The following mild abnormalities have been described in patients with chronic fatigue or ME:

- Reduction in aerobic work capacity – ability to perform sustained exercise. This has been shown by Dr Marrie and colleagues from Nova Scotia and Dr Riley and colleagues from Belfast, Northern Ireland. These changes, however, could be due, not only to an active viral infection, but to the loss of muscle enzymes which might occur because of nutritional factors.

- The presence of genetic material deposited by enteroviruses in the muscles of some patients with post-viral fatigue syndrome. This has been demonstrated by Dr Archard from London and Professor Behan from Glasgow. As many as 53 per cent of patients with fatigue had evidence of enteroviral genetic material in their muscles, compared with 15 per cent of a healthy population.

- A reduced rate at which muscles produce protein which is necessary for their repair and function. Researchers at King's College Hospital, London, led by Professor T.J. Peters, have shown reduced rates of protein manufacture in the thigh muscles of patients with ME compared with healthy people. Inactivity may have been responsible for some of this finding.

- Excessive accumulation of lactic acid has been observed in one patient with chronic fatigue syndrome. Lactic acid is produced in large amounts during exercise. If it accumulates, the muscles' metabolism becomes inefficient and muscle pain and cramps occur. This build up of lactic acid could also occur because of vitamin B1 (thiamin) deficiency or disease of muscle metabolism.

Nutritional factors, as we will see, have a profound effect on muscle function. Protein, most of the B group vitamins, magnesium and potassium are particularly important in influencing muscle metabolism and its ability to produce protein necessary for healthy functioning.

Evidence of a change in nervous system function

By now you probably are not going to be too surprised to learn that there may indeed be subtle changes in the nervous system in some patients with chronic fatigue syndrome or ME. It is known that some of the viruses that appear to be responsible for chronic fatigue syndrome can attack and persist in neurological (nerve) tissue, and by doing so may cause a change in nerve chemistry or function. A number of researchers have observed:

- Subtle changes on brain-wave tests (electro encephalogram – EEG) and changes in the transmission of electrical impulses along nerves that supply muscles. Again, it should be borne in mind that a variety of physical (including nutritional) factors and even psychological factors might influence the subtle workings of the nervous system.

• Changes in brain chemistry have also been observed. Dr Bakheit from Glasgow University in conjunction with the ever-active Professor Behan found, in a group of fifteen patients with post-viral fatigue syndrome, that the brain was particularly sensitive to a drug that stimulated the release of a hormone called prolactin. This suggested a change in body chemistry of a type different to that found in patients with pure depression. This might mean that there is an alteration in the function of the hypothalamus, the part of the brain which controls appetite, mood, the menstrual cycle in women, sleeping pattern and also hormone function.

To sum up

Essentially, we have evidence that a variable but high percentage of patients with chronic fatigue syndrome are different from the 'normal' healthy population. There is evidence in many patients of past infection with a variety of viruses in association with subtle changes in muscles, the nervous system and the immune system in a way that explains some of the symptoms experienced by those suffering from chronic fatigue syndrome and ME.

The evidence strongly supports the notion that there are numerous groups of patients, all of whom can be collectively diagnosed as having chronic fatigue syndrome. Those with evidence of muscle and nervous system changes would indeed qualify for the description myalgic encephalomyelitis (ME) particularly if immune disturbance is also present.

Unfortunately, at present the description of these abnormalities has not yet resulted in a broadly successful treatment approach. Therapies with drugs that stimulate the immune system have given mixed and usually disappointing results. In view of what is known about the influence of nutritional factors upon muscle function and immune system function, the existing evidence would suggest that this would be a fruitful area for exploration. Furthermore, a wide variety of both psychological and physical factors can influence immune function and again some of these aspects may well prove to be important in developing successful treatments.

4

Fatigue and continuing infection

Occasionally people visit the doctor because of fatigue when it is the most obvious symptom of a hidden active and treatable infection. This is distinct from fatigue that has been caused by a past infection, the acute phase of which lasted for a few weeks and then cleared leaving persistent fatigue, as in the case of myalgic encephalomyelitis. The purpose of this chapter is to describe briefly some of those possible infections so that they are not omitted from the assessment of someone with chronic fatigue. Something that may not seem relevant to you the patient could be the vital clue to the cause of your illness.

Most descriptions of chronic fatigue states include the presence of a low-level fever which may be present either occasionally or frequently. No study in recent times has documented the levels and ranges of temperatures that could be expected in those suffering from chronic fatigue. We just don't know. Until very recently we didn't even know what a normal temperature is. But more of that later.

This acceptance of a slight fever in chronic fatigue introduces the potential for overlooking an active hidden infection which is the cause of the fever and the fatigue. But a fever is not the only feature of a continuing infection. Your doctor will try to identify a likely infection from a range of possibilities by asking you relevant questions about the symptoms you have and whether you may have come into contact with any unusual or exotic organisms or infections.

First of all, a few words about deciding if there is a fever or not.

HAVE I GOT A FEVER?

I'm sorry for the technical details but the question of, 'Is there or is there not a fever?' is an extremely important one for patient and doctor alike. To answer it, it may be necessary to record the temperature several times a day for a week or two including those occasions when you feel hot, chilly or are sweating. Measuring and recording your temperature on a regular basis is a useful way to help your doctor assess and monitor your symptoms.

The previously assumed normal temperature of 37°C (98.6°F) has recently been shown to be a little too high and the new average is 36.8°C (98.6°F). There is also quite a considerable variation in temperature during the day, with the lowest levels being recorded in the early morning or on waking and the highest between 4 and 6p.m. This natural variation is on average 0.5°C (0.9°F) but can be as much as 1.3°C (2.3°F).

The upper limit for a normal temperature during the day for normal healthy adults is now considered to be 37.7°C, (100°F). However, the upper level for a normal temperature taken first thing in the morning before getting out of bed is 37.1°C (98.9°F) and temperatures above these levels should be considered to be abnormal.

All of these measurements should be made using thermometers placed under the tongue and according to the instructions. If the old-fashioned but accurate mercury thermometer is used it too should be placed under the tongue and left with the mouth closed for four minutes. Don't forget to shake down the thermometer before putting it into the mouth and don't clean it with hot or warm water as this will cause it to burst.

Here are some questions to help determine if you have a hidden active infection.

Questionnaire

- Do you have a fever – temperatures of 37.8°C (100°F) or above?

- Do you have any of the following symptoms which may signify a hidden localised infection:
    Pain on passing urine?
    Pain in the lower abdomen/pelvic region?
    Dental pain?
    Pain in the face?
    Earache or discharge from the ear?
    Chronic catarrh from the nose?
    A chronic cough with or without phlegm?
    Diarrhoea?
    Mucus or blood in the stools?
    Painful or swollen glands in the neck, armpits or groins?
    Pain and tenderness to touch in any part of the body excluding muscles?

- Have you ever had a chronic infection in the past,

especially a tropical illness or osteomyelitis (infection of the bone)?

- Within the year preceding the onset of your illness did you travel abroad to any tropical or sub-tropical countries including North America and Australia? If so did you experience any illness when abroad?

- Did (and do) you have any contact with wild animals including:
    Deer?
    Wild boar or pigs?
    Bears?
    Rodents?
    Reptiles?
    Parrots?
    Exotic animals?
    Cattle?

- Have you experienced any tick bites in association with any of the above animals?

- Are you a farmer, veterinary surgeon, abattoir worker or employed in other work that involves contact with cattle, poultry or animal products, e.g. raw meat, hides, etc.

- Have you had contact with puppies or cats, especially any who had recently given birth to kittens?

- Have you eaten any under-cooked meats, especially wild meats or lamb?

- Have you walked in forested areas where you might have been bitten by ticks?

- Have you eaten cheese or consumed other dairy products that might not have been pasteurised?

- Are you known to have heart disease with damaged or leaky heart valves or a heart murmur?

- Are you one of (or have you been a sexual partner of one of) the following risk groups for HIV:
    Homosexual men?
    Intravenous drug users?
    Haemophiliacs?
    A receiver of medical treatment involving injections or a blood transfusion in a Third World country?

- Have you lost weight with a fever during your illness?

- Do you know any one else with a similar illness beginning at approximately the same time as you, with whom you have had close contact or who has been in similar locations or engaged in similar activities as yourself?

Some of these rather strange and obscure questions may have aroused your interest. If your answer to any of these was positive then you should bring this to the attention of your doctor if you have not already done so. As you read the next few pages describing numerous infections that can cause fatigue, it will become clear how relevant these questions are.

SPECIFIC INFECTIONS

Now a few words about some of these hidden infections. Most are rare but some are quite common and have a reputation for being easily overlooked.

Bladder or kidney infection

This type of infection is commonly known as cystitis. It is rare in men but not infrequent in women and can occur silently. More usually it causes pain on passing water, an increased frequency of going to the toilet and smelly or cloudy urine. Diagnosis is by a simple urine test and treatment with antibiotics is highly successful.

Chronic sinus infection

Chronic catarrh from the nose or at the back of the throat, sometimes with headaches or pain in the face, are the main symptoms. An X-ray and examination will determine if this type of infection is present. It is helped by antibiotics, steam inhalations and if severe by surgery. Identification of possible allergies can also be important as they may be triggering the symptoms.

Hidden dental infection

This can be a cause of fever and malaise but should be detected by finding gum swelling, pain or tenderness on touching the teeth or changes on X-ray.

Gynaecological infection in women (pelvic inflammatory disease)

Hidden infection of the Fallopian tubes which join the ovaries to the uterus is a common health problem in women of reproductive age. It is commonly known as pelvic inflammatory disease and it is estimated that 15 per cent of women in the United States have had this infection by the age of thirty! The infection is often carried silently with acute episodes, characterised by abdominal pain, vaginal discharge and a fever. The infection may only show if special types of swabs are taken with great care. It is treated with a combination of two antibiotics which may need to be taken for several weeks. If not treated properly infertility may result.

Hidden sexual infection in men

Men, too, can have a similar infection to women which can cause pain on passing urine, a discharge from the end of the penis and discomfort at the base of the penis or underneath. It is often due to the same germs that causes pelvic inflammatory disease in women and again infection with these organisms sometimes called NSU – non-specific urethritis – can be a cause of fatigue usually with local symptoms.

Chest infections

These are usually obvious because of symptoms such as coughing with the production of phlegm. Smokers are more likely to suffer, but some people are predisposed to repeated chest or throat infections and this occasionally runs in a family.

Gastro-intestinal infections

The commonest of these include the echoviruses that have been strongly associated with the development of true myalgic encephalomyelitis. As well as this and a wide variety of other viruses and bacteria that can cause acute and short-lived diarrhoea, there are a number of different germs that can produce chronic bowel symptoms with fatigue as a main complaint.

Giardiasis   This is the term for infection by a parasitic organism called *giardia lamblia* that can produce either an acute or chronic bowel infection. It has been found increasingly frequently in Western countries and can now be caught in the US, UK or most European countries. It should be seriously considered in anyone with fatigue and bowel symptoms. Unfortunately, diagnosis can be very difficult as the organism does not always show in a stool sample.

Dr Leo Galland from the United States reported finding *giardia* in sixty-three of 218 patients who came to his practice complaining mainly of fatigue. However, the method he used to make the diagnosis was not one that is widely accepted. No similar survey has been undertaken in the UK and this work is definitely in need of repetition as Dr Galland reported a high degree of success with standard treatment with antibiotics. It would seem common sense to investigate the possibility of *giardia* infection if fatigue is accompanied by diarrhoea or abdominal pain.

Case History

Ben Church

Ben Church was a lively ten-year-old. He had been off school for six weeks because of occasional fevers and diarrhoea. This at first seemed like gastro-enteritis from which he had failed to recover fully.

Assessment by two paediatricians (doctors who special-ise in treating children) and his general practitioner had not revealed any serious disease and his mother wondered whether dietary problems might now be causing his symp-toms. Ben was clearly dejected and fed up with seeing so many doctors. It seemed likely that he might be having problems with certain foods including dairy products and I suggested that he try excluding these and a variety of other foods to see if this helped.

An old-fashioned treatment for patients with persistent diarrhoea after gastro-enteritis is to give supplements of vitamin B. Indeed there is evidence now that supplements of vitamin B may help recovery from acute diarrhoea when it occurs in children in underdeveloped countries. I thought I would check Ben's vitamin B3 level – nicotinamide – and to my surprise it was quite low. I phoned his mother and suggested he took some supplements of strong vitamin B complex and this together with the dietary changes resulted in considerable improvement, but he was not fully better as he was still running a temperature from time to time. An old GP of his then suggested that he might have infection with *giardia lamblia* even though his tests for this were negative. He took a three-day course of the antibiotic metronidazole. This resulted in a marked improvement and total clearance of his residual diarrhoea and feeling of ill-health.

Salmonella   This is an organism that typically produces acute and severe diarrhoea – food poisoning – and can occasionally cause a hidden chronic infection.

Amoebiasis   This is a parasite that can infest the gut and is caught almost exclusively in tropical countries. It can cause an acute or chronic illness characterised by diarrhoea, abdominal pain and malaise with or without a fever. It should be considered if you have been to south-east Asia, west and south Africa, Mexico and southern America.

Case History

Jack Minor

Jack Minor was an adventurer who liked to take off to far-flung corners of Asia for long periods. It was about a year previously that he had had a bout of amoebic dysentery when he was in India and this had responded well to antibiotic treatment. I saw him on his return six months later when he was working as a bus conductor. He was complaining of mild fatigue. He had no fever and his stools were loose only occasionally. General examination was normal as were routine blood tests, and a stool test showed no sign of a return of the amoebic dysentery or other parasites. I thought he might have developed a mild intolerance to milk sugar – lactose – or other foods and I suggested changes in his diet but this was of no real benefit. The fatigue continued but was not severe enough to cause him to take time off work.

I got a phone call from him a few days before he was due to go out to India again. His stools had become looser and he was passing two or three per day but without any blood. He didn't want to disrupt his trip to India so I suggested that he go to a clinic as soon as he arrived out there to see if he still had any amoebae in the stool. Indeed this was the case and it responded well to a course of antibiotics, this time combined with Indian herbal medicine! Occasionally infection with amoebae can produce chronic disease which may pass unnoticed for several years. This can sometimes spread to the liver. Occasionally it may be missed on one stool test and repeated stool tests are required.

Toxoplasmosis

This is an infection with an organism which is widely distributed throughout the world. In Western countries it is most often associated with the domestic cat. It is usually spread by contact with sheep, cats or new-born kittens which can be highly infectious. The infection is often silent with 10 per cent of ten-year-olds and 50 per cent of seventy-year-olds showing evidence of past infection. Infection is particularly common in France.

In most people who are infected only a very mild illness is experienced or none at all. However, some develop an illness which is virtually identical to glandular fever, with enlarged and painful glands in the neck or elsewhere, a sore throat, headache and fever. The illness may be prolonged for months with significant fatigue as a major feature. Infection during pregnancy is usually silent and of no consequence for the mother but can result in a miscarriage or severe abnormality in the baby. When pregnant, women should take care when handling cats, cat litter and raw meat. Beware the rare steak and hamburger. The germ is destroyed by hot water or cooking to a heat of 60°C (140°F).

Treatment of those with an active troublesome infection is with antibiotics; however, the symptoms may spontaneously improve.

Infection with parasites

There are a wide variety of parasitic infections which can produce illness in which fatigue (often, but not always with a fever) is a feature. Most of these are caught during travels to tropical or sub-tropical countries but some can be found closer to home in the Mediterranean, the Caribbean, North

America and Europe and should be actively considered in diagnosing patients with chronic fatigue. (This is the expert recommendation of the US committee which was convened to look at the problem of chronic fatigue.)

The main symptoms of most of these parasitic infections include:

- Weight loss.
- Diarrhoea.
- Nutritional deficiencies.
- Liver inflammation.
- Allergic reactions especially skin rashes.
- Epilepsy or other neurological problems.
- Loss of vision.
- Muscle pains.
- Cough and lung problems.
- Bowel and bladder problems.

Diagnosis is usually considered when the patient has a history of foreign travel; if there has been exposure to a possible source of infection, e.g. contaminated water, raw or under-cooked wild meat or fish; a combination of the above symptoms; or if the patient's blood tests show an increase in the level of white cells called eosinophils.

This blood abnormality can also be caused by an allergy and has been found to occur in five out of 200 patients in a British report by Dr Sharpe and colleagues from Oxford. It is likely that you would be referred for specialist assessment by a physician experienced in tropical diseases. Thankfully, there are many effective treatments.

Tuberculosis

This bacterial infection was once the scourge of both the deprived and the wealthy during the last century; TB has never been eradicated and recent statistics have shown a small but alarming rise in the UK and the USA. This disease is a slowly progressive lung infection that particularly affects alcoholics, vagrants and also urban dwelling immigrants (especially strict vegans). However, one-off cases do occur in other sections of the community. Fever, weight loss, night sweats, cough and a severe fatigue are typical symptoms. TB can also infect the bone, bowels, nervous system and occasionally the first symptom seen by a doctor is enlarged neck glands. Cases sometimes occur in people who have had contact with any of the above groups. Response to prolonged antibiotic treatment is usually good but recovery can be slow.

Heart valve infection

Infection of the valves of the heart is a serious and potentially fatal illness which can be easily overlooked. The elderly and those with damaged and leaky heart valves are at risk of bacteria settling on the heart valves from the bloodstream. Fever, which may only be slight at first, is accompanied by a host of other problems. Several weeks or months may pass before the diagnosis is obvious. Prompt treatment with antibiotics is essential, otherwise death may result which, sadly, is something I have witnessed.

Brucellosis

This is a rare but classic infective cause of chronic fatigue and sometimes depression. The organism, a bacterium, is found in cattle and is passed to humans by the consumption of unpasteurised milk products or by close contact with infected cows, sheep, goats or pigs as in the case of farmers, veterinary surgeons and abattoir workers.

Though eradicated from most parts of the developed world it can still occasionally occur in the United Kingdom; North, Central and South America; Australia and New Zealand; Mediterranean countries; the Middle and Far East.

Infection produces either an acute condition similar to a severe bout of flu or a chronic illness which can be hard to diagnose as it causes fatigue worsened by effort, muscular aches and pains, an increased need for sleep, sweats and either a slight or no fever. This picture may also be easily attributed to other ills or even depression. Diagnosis is only by blood tests and successful treatment requires the long-term use of antibiotics.

Lyme disease

This is a 'new' infection which has only been recognised for the last decade. It was once thought to be confined to the United States from where the first instances were reported but now it is found in the United Kingdom and because the course of the infection can be variable and slow it can easily be confused with a post-viral fatigue state.

Lyme disease is caused by an organism that rejoices in the name *borrelia burgdorferi*. The bite of a tick transmits the bacteria from its reservoir in deer to man. The initial reaction is a rash spreading out from the bite and this can be accompanied by fever, malaise and gland enlargement. There then follows a chronic phase when fatigue, joint pains and swellings, and a variety of neurological problems including headaches, weakness, numbness and tingling occur.

Diagnosis can be difficult as the initial illness may pass unnoticed or the tick bite is not remembered. It has been known to masquerade as chronic fatigue syndrome and

must now be seriously considered as a possible treatable
infective cause. More cases are likely to be reported in the
coming years. It responds well to antibiotic treatment
which occasionally needs to be prolonged.

Fungal infections

This is not about common infections with Candida or any
of the many other minor fungal infections that mainly
cause superficial infections of the skin, nails, hair, mouth or
vagina. In addition to these there are some rare and serious
fungal infections which mainly occur in North, Central and
South America, Africa, Asia and occasionally in Europe.
They produce acute or chronic infections often affecting
the lungs or skin. They are very rare but should be
considered in those who have travelled abroad.

Candida

See separate section pages 175–186.

HIV infection (Human Immunodeficiency Virus)

This now has to be considered in the diagnosis of those
with chronic fatigue. The HIV virus itself can directly cause
substantial ill-health because of its effects on the body,
especially the immune system, and because it weakens the
natural defence systems it leaves the body open to unusual
and often chronic infections.

There is no need for a long discourse on HIV infection
and its progress to the Acquired Immune Deficiency
Syndrome (AIDS). It is prudent to point out the main risk
groups for this pernicious infection, though this may not
identify all those who have contracted the virus.

Although large sections of the heterosexual community are infected in some parts of the developing world, in western countries the main at-risk groups include:

- Homosexual men.
- Intravenous drug users.
- Haemophiliacs.
- Those who have received contaminated blood products, organs or injections with contaminated equipment.
- Sexual partners of any of the above.
- Children born to mothers who themselves are HIV positive.

Cases of hidden or latent infection may be present in certain heterosexual communities.

Diagnosis is easily made by a blood test though this can, on occasion, be misleading. A falsely positive result can be obtained in some conditions, and more seriously those who have just acquired the virus and are carrying it may not test positive until three months have elapsed.

Chronic hepatitis

Certain types of viral infections of the liver – hepatitis – can lead to chronic illness where fatigue may be an early feature. These virus infections are found mainly in tropical or sub-tropical climes and cause an acute or silent infection which, in a small percentage of people, leads to a slow and sometimes progressive illness. Diagnosis is suggested by finding slightly abnormal liver tests and then evidence of the virus itself. Many infections resolve spontaneously but some sufferers require medical treatment.

Finally it should be remembered that a variety of non-infective illnesses can cause a fever as well as fatigue. This includes any disease where there is a lot of inflammation as in certain types of arthritis and even vitamin B12 deficiency.

WHAT TO DO IF ANY OF THE ABOVE
APPLIES TO YOU

If, while reading this chapter, some of the questions in the first part applied to you *and* you have a fever (a temperature of 37.8°C (100°F) or above, then you should immediately bring this to the attention of your doctor if you have not done so already.

Virtually all of the conditions above cause ill-health lasting for weeks or months, and not just fever for a few days which then settles completely.

WHAT TO DO IF NONE OF THE ABOVE
APPLIES TO YOU

This should be the situation in 99 per cent or more of readers. Your doctor has probably already considered all of the above conditions that are relevant, and if you have seen a medical specialist then tests may have already been performed that might detect the more common problems.

Hopefully this will reassure you that this aspect of your care has been looked at. Thus time can be more usefully spent on other aspects of your healthcare and on constructive ways in which recovery from fatigue can be achieved.

5

Fatigue caused by physical illness

As we have seen, there are a number of physical causes for fatigue. In this chapter, I am going to consider non-infective illnesses that may cause fatigue. People going to their doctors with most of these conditions also have a wide variety of other distinguishing symptoms, or other features that allow them to be easily and clearly identified. Unfortunately, many or all can start with fatigue in their early stages, which presents the ultimate challenge for the busy physician.

One of the purposes of this chapter is to help share that burden of responsibility by informing you about some of these illnesses so that you can help your doctor decide whether further assessment for one of the following conditions is necessary.

Before I launch into what may be regarded as the ultimate hypochondriac's checklist there is a questionnaire for you to complete. If, after you have done this, you feel that none of the questions apply, then you need not claw your way through the most technical chapter in this book.

If, however, one or more of the questions apply, discuss this with your doctor if you have not done so already.

Questionnaire

1. Have you lost or gained weight recently without changing your diet?
2. Do you have a cough with or without phlegm?
3. Do you experience wheezing or shortness of breath at rest or on modest exertion?
4. Have you experienced chest pains or palpitations (rapid or irregular heart beats)?
5. When walking, do you experience pains in the calf muscles or feet that are quickly relieved by rest?
6. Have you noticed that you are passing more urine than usual? And is it very frothy, painful to pass, discoloured or does it contain blood?
7. Have you experienced a change in your normal bowel habit, developed constipation, diarrhoea or seen blood or a darkening of your stools?
8. Has your skin become very itchy or have you developed a skin rash or easy bruising?
9. Have you become intolerant of very hot or cold weather?
10. For women – have your periods become very heavy, light, infrequent or irregular?
11. Do you or others around you think that your facial appearance changed since your illness began?
12. Have the size of your feet or hands increased and have you noticed gaps developing between your teeth or your dentures not fitting well?
13. Have you noticed a significant loss of libido not related to stress?

14. Have you been experiencing unexplained persistent pains?

15. Have you noticed any loss or disturbance of vision, pain in the eyes or drooping of the eyelids?

16. Have you experienced any of the following:
    • Persistent numbness or tingling?
    • Muscle wasting?
    • Muscle twitches?
    • Tremors or shakes of the hands?
    • Loss of balance or giddiness?

17. Have you developed enlarged glands or unexplained lumps?

18. Have any of your joints been painful and either swollen, warm or red?

19. Do you experience *severe* pain or weakness in your muscles during or shortly after exercise? If so does rest bring rapid relief?

20. Does anyone in your family have similar health problems or a disease affecting the muscles or nerves?

21. Does anyone in the family have:
    • Diabetes?
    • Thyroid disease?
    • Other hormonal problems?
    • Rheumatoid arthritis?
    • Coeliac disease?
    • Heart disease?
    • Lung disease?
    • Liver disease?
    • Other serious health problems?

22. Have you experienced recent onset of severe or unusual headaches, blackouts or giddy spells?

23. Has your fatigue or other symptoms come on since starting or changing the type or dosage of a prescribed drug?

24. Do you consume more than six units of alcohol per day (four if you are a woman), or does drinking alcohol greatly aggravate the symptoms of muscle pain or fatigue?
25. Does eating sugar, sweet foods, fruit or meat greatly aggravate any of your symptoms?

THE HEALTHY FUNCTIONING OF THE BODY

To better understand some of the important physical conditions which are described in the following pages, here are a few words about the overall function of the body. Without it, it may be easy to become a little confused.

The healthy functioning of the body is determined by two main categories of factors – genetic and environmental.

Genetic

By genetic we mean the inherited material that makes up the centre or nucleus of the body's cells and determines the type of metabolism that we have. A wide range of variations and abnormalities of metabolism are known, and these can cause either mild or serious disturbances of health which may be evident at birth or not until middle or even old age. Many genetically determined ills are also greatly influenced by environmental factors such as diet, medical drugs or infections.

Environmental

A whole host of environmental factors potentially influence both the structure and function of tissues. This includes outside factors such as infecting organisms, the supply of essential nutrients, the presence of toxins, and subtle unspecified factors that may determine the rate at which wear and tear take place in the tissues. The immune system may be particularly susceptible to environmental factors.

The body can be imagined as a smooth-running, brilliantly designed, flexible engine. Unlike mechanical engines, it is built with a huge margin of error. In other words, it is built to work even when diseased. It has many fail-safe mechanisms which means that instead of packing up at the first sign of problems, it carries on functioning – but at the expense of a loss of efficiency. Typically, humans thrive on challenge, and our bodies are robust enough to survive the initial challenge of many genetically and environmentally determined illnesses. Consequently we have the time to apply our minds and resources to the problem of recovery.

For ease of understanding, I have broken down the relevant physical illnesses and conditions into different groups to help you assess whether they may apply to you. For each condition or group of ills I have identified some of the risk factors – such as family history and previous health problems – that might serve as a pointer to diagnosis. Typical symptoms of a condition are given and a brief outline of its effects on health.

PHYSICAL CONDITIONS THAT CAUSE FATIGUE

By now, you will probably appreciate that there are a large number of medical conditions that can cause fatigue. The information that follows is taken from many important publications on fatigue, particularly that by Dr Gary P. Holmes and colleagues from the Center for Disease Control in Atlanta, Georgia, USA. Their publication, 'Chronic Fatigue Syndrome: A working case definition', appeared in the *Annals of Internal Medicine* (1988) and gives a long list of the medical conditions which can cause fatigue and should be investigated by 'thorough evaluation based on history, physical examination and appropriate laboratory findings'.

In the United Kingdom, Dr Peter O. Behan, Professor of Neurology at the University Department of Neurology, Southern General Hospital, Glasgow, Scotland, also produced an excellent booklet *Diagnostic and Clinical Guidelines for Doctors* for the Myalgic Encephalomyelitis Association, and it too contains much pertinent advice on the physical illnesses that can be confused with myalgic encephalomyelitis. The remaining information is taken from standard medical texts.

Lung disease

This has occasionally been recorded in patients with fatigue. Diagnosis should be relatively easy and suggested by symptoms such as shortness of breath, wheezing or coughing. Asthma is the most likely lung condition, but other allergic or inflammatory lung conditions are also possible. Physical examination, simple blood tests and chest X-rays should detect most lung problems.

Heart disease

Similarly, some types of heart disease could begin with fatigue. Most usually, symptoms of shortness of breath on exercise or at rest, chest pains on exercise, ankle swelling or palpitations would be present, but these may not always be obvious.

Most fatigue and shortness of breath caused by heart disease improves, partially at least, with a few minutes of rest and this may be an important clue. Examination, chest X-ray and electrocardiogram (ECG-EKG) would rapidly lead to a diagnosis. If there is a family history of heart disease, particularly starting at a young age, then this should increase suspicion that there is an underlying heart problem. Very occasionally heart disease can follow a viral infection.

Case History

Arthur Jones

Arthur Jones was a robust fifty-five-year-old landscape gardener and casual labourer. His main complaints were episodes of fatigue and shortness of breath. Usually after his ten minutes' brisk walk to work he would have to sit or lie down. During the recovery he would sweat profusely with a rapid heartbeat. He had also noticed periods when he would have to pass urine more often, and now got up eight or nine times at night. Apparently, his general practitioner had found little wrong with him and suggested supplements of potassium which seemed to have helped slightly.

When I saw him, however, his heart rate was 144 per minute. Urgent referral to a heart specialist revealed that he had an abnormal heart rhythm which was probably intermittent and caused his fatigue, shortness of breath, and an increased need to go to the toilet. Treatment by his specialist with some simple drugs resulted in marked improvement.

Again, an intermittent heart rhythm can manifest itself

with sporadic fatigue. Modern methods of diagnosis with ECG, EKG and twenty-four-hour monitoring can now be undertaken which should allow detection of even the most difficult cases.

Kidney disease

Kidney failure is a possible cause of fatigue which should be easily detected. Kidney failure can cause anaemia, and disturbance in the body's balance of the minerals sodium and potassium will disrupt muscle function. This can occur quite silently especially in older people and is most likely in those with a history of diabetes, high blood pressure, urine infections or other waterwork problems. Routine blood and urine tests will detect these problems.

Diseases of the bowel

Serious bowel conditions where there is considerable inflammation of the bowel, such as Crohn's disease and ulcerative colitis, are likely to begin with diarrhoea, abdominal pain and blood in the stools before fatigue develops.

Coeliac disease, a condition in which there is a marked allergy to gluten (a protein in wheat, oat, barley and rye) can first appear in many ways. Because it prevents the intestines absorbing food efficiently, it most usually causes weight loss, anaemia caused by lack of iron and folic acid, and abdominal bloating and distention. Fatigue may be a prominent and sometimes early feature. Coeliac disease should not be confused with mild forms of gluten intolerance, which may cause minor bowel symptoms and possibly fatigue. There is more on this subject in Chapter 12 on Fatigue and Allergy (pages 165–74). Fatigue can sometimes

be the first signs of certain rare disorders of the bowel
before the abdominal symptoms develop.

Case History

Alistair MacMichael

Alistair was a friend I had known for several years who
had no love of doctors. He thought he had been having
repeated bouts of flu over the preceding year with night
sweats but no fever, and fatigue. He had lost four to five
pounds in weight, despite a hearty appetite, but had no
serious symptoms. His one bad habit was smoking (twenty
to thirty cigarettes per day).

The only abnormality on examination was a slight
enlargement of his liver and enlargement of the spleen (a
large gland in the abdomen rather like a giant lymph node).
This suggested that something more serious than flu was
going on. His blood test showed a mild anaemia (see
Chapter 7 on Fatigue and Iron). Clearly something was
going on and I referred him to chest specialists, but several
weeks of very thorough investigations did not lead to any
diagnosis.

He improved slightly, left hospital and started to go back
to work. A few weeks later he developed a fever, abdominal bloating and he was running a temperature. The only
area still to be explored was his bowel and he went to see
a specialist gastro-enterologist. Further investigations
revealed that he had a very rare gastro-intestinal infection
– Whipple's disease – which responded very well to
prolonged treatment with antibiotics. It seemed likely that
this infection had been gradually building up over a period
of eighteen months or longer.

Liver disease

The liver is involved in many of the body's metabolic functions. Jaundice – yellow discolouration of the skin and eyes – is the most obvious sign of liver problems, but sometimes the gradual onset of fatigue can be the first indication of a liver condition. Minor abnormalities on blood/liver function tests are found not infrequently in some people with chronic fatigue and occasionally in the normal population. They may be due to alcohol excess; recovery from a viral infection e.g. glandular fever virus; an active virus infection – which may need treatment; or actual diseases of the liver or metabolism.

Symptoms, such as fatigue or skin itching, heavy periods, perhaps with hysterectomy, may all be clues to an underlying liver problem.

Blood tests which show liver function should be performed routinely in people with serious fatigue and minor changes in liver function should be followed up carefully.

Case History

Deborah Singleton

Deborah Singleton was referred to me by her general practitioner because of a continuing history of fatigue, weight gain and mild memory impairment. She had been reading up about thyroid disease and felt certain that her thyroid was under-active. Thyroid function tests were, however, quite normal. As a precaution, I ran some routine blood tests and this showed a minor liver abnormality. I suggested that this was repeated and further tests were performed a month or two later. These in fact revealed that she had a mild and early liver disease – primary biliary cirrhosis – which mainly affects middle-aged women. She was referred to a liver specialist as careful assessment and monitoring is required. A weight-reducing diet, combined with some multivitamins to make sure that her intake of these was adequate, resulted in a modest improvement in her fatigue. She also felt reassured that she had been thoroughly assessed.

Hormonal problems

Hormones are substances produced in small quantities by one cell which are excreted into the bloodstream. They pass to another or target tissue, where they stimulate a change in metabolism or function in that tissue. They have wide ranging and powerful effects. Most of us, I am sure, are familiar with hormones in relation to the ovaries in women and the testicles in men and how they affect sexual function. There is also a wide range of other hormones produced by the thyroid and parathyroid glands in the neck, the adrenal glands in the abdomen, and the pituitary gland at the base of the brain. As hormonal problems are such an important cause of fatigue, I will consider these glands individually.

Thyroid disease

The thyroid gland produces the hormone thyroxine which acts as a stimulus to the metabolism of all cells of the body. A lack of thyroxine leads to a slowing down in the body's level of activity and an increase results in a speeding up. It is rather like the accelerator pedal in a car. Thyroid disease is very common, affecting perhaps 1 per cent of the population. It is common enough, and serious enough, for all newborn babies to be screened for thyroid disease.

Many elderly patients, especially those being admitted to hospital, are also often screened as routine. Thyroid assessment should be part of the routine examination of many patients with severe fatigue. The risks for thyroid disease are increased if family members have thyroid problems.

An over-active thyroid As you may imagine, this results in increased pulse rate, increased appetite, weight loss, sweating, palpitations, or rapid heart rate. Sometimes people suffer with vomiting and diarrhoea as well.

An under-active thyroid This produces the opposite symptoms: weight gain, an intolerance to cold, lethargy, muscular aches and pains, and a pale pasty complexion. Fatigue is also a common feature. Severe cases are less common as doctors are now more aware of under-activity of the thyroid and because tests for thyroid function have improved remarkably over the last twenty years. Occasionally, fatigue or depression and mental changes may be the main or only features. The most sensitive test measures TSH – thyroid stimulating hormone – which is often used as a useful screening test for patients with thyroid problems.

Case History

June Patrick

June admitted at the start that her problems were stress related. She had actually experienced a mild stroke at the age of forty, two years before she came to see me. Since then she had had disturbed sleep, weight gain of two stones and mood swings. Her energy level was low. She had tried taking a wide variety of vitamin and mineral supplements, and also an American preparation that included adrenal and thyroid gland extract!

I asked her to come back six weeks after she had come off all her previous treatments so that I could make a better assessment as to what was going on. I recommended a healthy nutrient-rich, weight-reducing diet. At her second consultation her blood tests showed a mildly under-active thyroid, which was confirmed on a repeat test a further six weeks later. Her thyroid was indeed mildly under-active and in need of treatment. Treatment with a small dose of thyroid hormone replacement and a weight-loss diet improved her energy level greatly.

Self-administering extracts of thyroid and adrenal glands is inadvisable because it is unlikely that the patient will be able to treat themselves correctly (the dose strength in different tablets can vary and it could easily cause side-effects), and using them may mask more serious illness.

Disease of the parathyroid glands

The parathyroid glands are four match-head sized glands found in the neck which are embedded in the back of the thyroid gland itself (*para* is Latin for 'at the side of'). They produce a hormone that has a profound effect upon calcium levels in the blood. Like the thyroid glands, they can be either over- or under-active. Over-activity of the glands causes an increase in blood calcium which may result in aches and pains, abdominal pains, high blood pressure, mental changes, kidney stones and fatigue. Weight loss, increasing thirst and depression may also be features.

A lack of parathyroid gland hormone occurs when they

are removed by accident during surgery on the thyroid gland or when they just gradually stop functioning. A low blood calcium, sometimes associated with muscle spasms, easy fatigue, and tingling in the arms and legs, may develop. Patients with a history of thyroid operations some twenty or thirty years ago before the importance of the parathyroid glands was fully realised may be particularly at risk.

Measurement of blood calcium level, part of the routine examination for the majority of fatigued patients, will detect these problems.

Case History

Melonie Griffiths

Melonie Griffiths was a thirty-two-year-old housewife with two children. For over ten years she had been known to have coeliac disease, a severe allergy to gluten, and had been very carefully avoiding all foods containing wheat, oats, barley and rye. In the last year, however, she had begun to develop intense muscle spasms and fatigue, and had lost 5 kilos (11 lbs) in weight. Her doctor had been prudent enough to run some tests which showed she had a high level of blood calcium (3.2 millimols per litre which was some 20 per cent above normal). Initially, her doctor had not believed the result, and had repeated the test on two occasions before she finally came to see me. I was alarmed by her calcium results too. A very high blood calcium is a serious condition. The most likely diagnosis was excess production of parathyroid hormone. I quickly got in touch with the local specialist and she was admitted under his care the next day, before being referred on to a teaching hospital for removal of an enlarged and over-enthusiastic parathyroid gland. Within six weeks of the operation she had made an almost complete recovery from her muscle spasms and fatigue, and she had begun to regain her weight.

Case History

Winifred Piggott

Winifred Piggott was a chirpy seventy-six-year-old who had been troubled by some six upper respiratory tract infections – coughs and colds – in the preceding year. She had also had long-standing irritable bowel syndrome, modest fatigue and some muscular aches and pains which, she asserted, improved whenever she took multivitamins and calcium tablets. The only health problem she had ever had was an enlarged thyroid gland which had been operated on thirty years previously. She had been treated with thyroid hormone since then and her thyroid tests were always satisfactory. Examination was normal enough and there was no evidence of anaemia or disturbance of liver function. The level of calcium in the blood was modestly reduced, almost certainly as a result of the loss of her parathyroid glands at the time of her thyroid operation thirty years previously.

She was placed on long-term calcium supplementation and this brought her blood calcium levels up into the normal range. To make sure that this was the right kind of treatment she was also checked by a specialist in calcium metabolism.

Since then she has remained very well taking her supplements of calcium and multivitamins on a regular basis.

The adrenal glands

The adrenal glands are two small glands which sit on top of or adjacent to the kidneys. They produce several hormones. An excess of adrenalin and its related hormone noradrenalin (which are known in North America as epinephrine and norepinephrine) result in high blood pressure, increased pulse rate and a picture similar to that of either an over-active thyroid or mild diabetes. Headaches, anxiety and a fluctuating blood pressure are characteristic features of this rare condition. Fatigue can again be a feature.

Case History

Diana Lightman

Fatigue wasn't Diana's main complaint; she had actually grown used to it. Coeliac disease had been diagnosed several years earlier, and she had resigned herself to always being slightly under-weight and tired. Recent tests had also shown that she had osteoporosis – thinning of the bones – and at the age of forty-seven she felt she should do something about this. She did not tolerate hormone replacement therapy (HRT) very well and I was concerned to find that she had very high blood pressure and headaches, especially as tests two years ago had not revealed any obvious cause for this. The physician who was monitoring her quickly repeated some of her earlier tests and found them now to be abnormal. The results suggested an adrenalin-producing tumour of the adrenal gland. This was the cause of her high blood pressure and headaches. A successful operation resulted in marked improvement in her blood pressure and general well-being.

She was now in a better position to tolerate her hormone

replacement therapy and other treatments to control her osteoporosis.

An excess of another hormone, cortisone, causes a condition called Cushing's syndrome, named after a famous American physician. Weight gain, a plump, rounded face with red cheeks, high blood pressure, stretch marks and muscle thinning with fatigue and weakness are all characteristic features. The same picture can occur when high doses of cortisone or other steroids are used in the treatment of allergic conditions or other diseases. Fatigue in conjunction with high blood pressure and weight gain around the abdomen should prompt consideration of this rare condition.

The near opposite condition to Cushing's syndrome is Addison's disease, this time named after a famous English physician from the last century. It too is a rare but important cause of fatigue which can develop slowly over months and years. Weight loss, poor appetite, salt craving, fatigue, and giddiness on standing up due to low blood pressure are the main features. Often there is a low level of the mineral potassium in the blood and low blood sugar. The response to treatment with cortisone and other hormones is dramatic.

Case History

Cecily Jones

Cecily was a twenty-nine-year-old woman who worked for a patent agent. She had only been unwell for the previous year following a series of minor colds which led to chronic fatigue. It was hard to imagine that such profound fatigue had followed such minor infections, and tests performed by a local specialist had been completely normal. She then came to see me for dietary advice, but there did not seem to be any problems there. Advice to eat even more healthily and try taking multivitamins was the best I could offer, but was of no benefit to her. As she had just split up with her boyfriend and had to move house as a result, I, and even she, was beginning to suspect that emotional factors were mainly to blame.

The only point of concern was that she had lost 3 kilos (6½lbs) in weight, which she could ill afford to lose as she only weighed 46 kilos (100 lbs). Her fatigue worsened so further investigations were arranged by her general practitioner and her original specialist. This revealed a fall in her blood potassium level. Her blood pressure was also low and this gave a clue that she might have Addison's disease – an under-active adrenal gland – which was indeed the case. There was a dramatic response to treatment with steroid replacement therapy and she made a full recovery.

Disease of the pituitary gland

The pituitary gland is the very important gland at the base of the brain which can be likened to the conductor of the hormonal orchestra. It controls the thyroid and adrenal glands and produces another hormone – growth hormone.

Abnormal functioning of the pituitary can result in a mixture of the hormonal problems described above.

An excess production of growth hormone by the pituitary can also occur, resulting in an excessive increase in height in children and variety of problems including muscle weakness and fatigue in adults. Other features which develop very slowly and serve as clues to this rare problem are: enlargement of the hands and feet resulting in bigger shoe and glove sizes, changes in facial appearance with a thickening of the lips and enlargement of the tongue, increasing gaps between the teeth or poorly fitting dentures, headache, arthritis and backache.

Diabetes mellitus

Diabetes mellitus is the proper and full term for 'diabetes'. In ancient Greek it means excessive passage of sweet urine. This characteristic feature is accompanied by an increased thirst, weight loss and malaise. In those whose diabetes starts when they are young (under the age of forty) there is usually a lack of the hormone insulin which is produced by the pancreas. Insulin's function is to assist the transport of sugar (glucose) from the bloodstream into the cells where it can be used as a source of energy. If the pancreas fails to produce enough insulin, it must be given by injection.

Diabetes beginning in later life is usually less severe and is not due to a lack of insulin but a reduction in the tissues' response to normal or even high amounts of insulin in the blood.

Fatigue can be caused by undiagnosed diabetes because of the disturbance in metabolism that occurs with raised blood-sugar levels. Many older people, especially those who are over-weight, may have mild diabetes without any typical symptoms. A simple urine and blood test will normally detect this and should be performed routinely. Treatment by diet, insulin injections or drugs is very successful.

Diseases of metabolism

There is also a collection of rare conditions that cause a disturbance in the metabolism – chemical processing – of certain substances such as sugars or proteins. The more usual and severe forms appear shortly after birth or in childhood, but milder forms do exist and may not be diagnosed until adult life. A wide variety of symptoms including headaches, abdominal pains, mental symptoms, fatigue, muscle pains and other features of ill-health are experienced. These symptoms are worsened or perhaps only occur when certain foods like sugar, fruits, sweets or protein-rich foods or certain drugs are consumed. They should be suspected if symptoms improve when fasting; if other members of the family have similar symptoms that are influenced by similar dietary habits; or if there has been a history of severe unexplained illness or death of a brother or sister in childhood.

Case History

Hilary Goldsack

Hilary's referral letter from her family doctor said it all: 'She has seen nine specialists in five years, can you help?' Her fatigue was her main complaint, but alas not her only one. Irregular periods and menstrual difficulties, nausea, poor appetite, abdominal symptoms, muscular aches and pains, headaches and depression were just some of the other complaints on her checklist. After a long and none too easy consultation, I too was mystified as to why she should have these symptoms and why they should vary so much from day to day. There were, however, a few curious little clues. She said she felt better when she didn't eat anything at all; her brother never ate sweets and had never eaten them as a child; a sister of hers had died at the age of three weeks because of 'gastro-enteritis'; and she herself had never been sporty at school. I had been fortunate enough to read of and see a similar case before.

A rare disturbance in metabolism involving fructose – fruit sugar which is derived from fruits and some vegetables – and sucrose – table sugar – can produce this complaint. Detailed metabolic assessment revealed that Diana had hereditary fructose intolerance. This genetically acquired condition is characterised by a variety of abdominal symptoms, mild fatigue and an aversion to sweets and sweet foods. It is likely that her sister, who died at the age of three weeks, and her brother also had this metabolic problem which can indeed be fatal in childhood.

She also had evidence of marked vitamin B1 (thiamin) and magnesium deficiencies, correction of which, together with changing her diet to exclude all sources of fructose, resulted in considerable improvement. Her menstrual difficulties required hormone treatment which was well tolerated.

Hereditary fructose intolerance is a rare condition occurring in one in every 20,000 of the normal population. If this book is a bestseller, a few readers may make a self-diagnosis of this condition, which, of course, will require careful confirmation by a specialist.

Cancer

Unfortunately fatigue may occasionally be the first sign of cancer and this should be borne in mind, especially in older patients. The fatigue can be due to an associated anaemia – lack of blood – or because of disturbances in the metabolism which will become evident from blood tests.

Case History

Barry Flowers

I didn't believe Mr Flowers for a minute when he said he had ME. Unfortunately, this was the diagnosis he had been given by his family doctor, but his ghastly pale appearance suggested that there was something else wrong. His low energy level, poor memory, fatigue and increasing shortness of breath had come on gradually over the preceding year and made him feel all of his seventy-four years.

Examination showed that he was very anaemic with signs that suggested he had mild vitamin C deficiency. Blood tests confirmed his anaemia with a haemoglobin level of 6.7 grams (half the expected level) and the lack of vitamin C.

Nutritional supplements alone were not, however, going to be the answer to his problem. Urgent referral to the hospital revealed the cause of his anaemia – cancer of the colon, which fortunately was found before it had a chance to spread. He made an excellent recovery from his operation before which he was given a course of strong multivitamins from the hospital, and he has remained well since.

Careful examination, routine blood tests and X-rays will detect most types of cancer. However, if fatigue persists particularly in association with weight loss, loss of appetite, pain or other unexplained symptoms then a reassessment should be undertaken.

Blood disorders

Certain blood conditions can cause mild anaemia which may not respond to treatment with iron or vitamins. This again should be detected by standard blood tests. Symptoms such as repeated infections, easy bruising, prolonged bleeding or excessively heavy periods may be due to such a blood disorder which in turn may be the root cause of the symptoms of fatigue.

Arthritis and inflammatory conditions

These conditions are included because muscular and joint aches and pains are a feature of true post-viral fatigue states and, of course, may be caused by other illnesses. An important point of difference is that if there is joint swelling or redness then an underlying form of arthritis is likely. This can occasionally follow on from certain viral infections and other conditions including glandular fever, German measles and some types of gastro-enteritis. In these cases there should be some clue from the patient's medical history.

Rheumatoid arthritis is not usually a crippling disease. It often occurs as a mild arthritis with a few swollen and painful joints, muscular aches and mild fatigue. Just occasionally it can be triggered by a viral infection and also can be caused or worsened by a true food allergy. It is indeed a common and 'versatile' condition.

Case History

Mavis Dance

Mavis was a forty-one-year-old factory worker whose main complaints were fatigue and aches and pains for six months. Over the last few weeks the aches and pains had become worse, now with slight swelling and pain in some of the knuckle joints of both hands. I thought she might have an early mild arthritis. Indeed, the tests for rheumatoid arthritis were positive and other routine tests for anaemia, kidney and liver function were quite satisfactory. She didn't want to take standard painkilling drugs so I suggested an exclusion diet. When she followed this strictly, there was a substantial reduction in her pain. When she broke the diet, however, there was initially no adverse effects, but after a week or so the pains returned. After careful trial and error over several months, it appeared that the pains were worse after drinking wine and eating wheat. Long-term avoidance of alcohol, yeast and gluten-containing cereals (wheat, oat, barley and rye) resulted in a 75 per cent reduction in her pain. She was able to return to full-time work.

Sometimes early rheumatoid arthritis may occur with fatigue as one of its earliest symptoms, particularly in association with muscular and joint pains. Rheumatoid arthritis and other related forms of arthritis should be considered in anyone with fatigue, joint pains and swelling especially if a variety of diverse problems is also present, including: skin rashes, especially on the face; circulation problems; fever; weight loss; chest, nose or throat symptoms; and other persistent problems affecting the heart, bowels, nervous system, eyes and kidneys. These conditions, known as auto-immune diseases because the body's immune system 'attacks' joints and muscles, often cause arthritis or muscular pains together with the wide variety of symptoms of ill-health described above. Sophisticated blood tests will often make the diagnosis and they usually respond well to expert drug treatment.

The wear and tear arthritis of older people – osteoarthritis – which often affects the hands, hips, knees and ankles is not itself a cause of fatigue.

Case History

Miranda Payne

Miranda Payne was a forty-three-year-old woman with many health problems. Fatigue was the main problem she wanted help with, but she generally had had more than her fair share of ills. Despite her age of forty-three, osteoporosis – thinning of the bones – had recently been diagnosed, she had just had an operation to remove part of her stomach because of an ulcer, she had a long history of low grade arthritis and back pain, eye inflammation and bowel problems, with constipation.

No drug therapy had been very successful, but she still required treatment with low doses of steroids for her eye problems, plus oestrogen and calcium for her osteoporosis. When she mentioned that she had had five miscarriages, I felt that there had to be something else going on to account for all these diverse problems. Indeed, she was being seen by five different specialists. Other blood tests indicated that she had an auto-immune condition where her immune system produced antibodies that were attacking different parts of her body. This is a very rare type (caused by anticardiolipin antibodies) which is known to cause recurrent miscarriages or recurrent blood clots. Referral to a specialist with expertise in this condition resulted in a review of her drug treatment. A calcium-rich, nutritious diet was also recommended to help her osteoporosis and fatigue. The changes helped her fatigue and arthritis. Fatigue, arthritis and a wide variety of other medical complaints may therefore indicate rare and sometimes chronic auto-immune conditions and they should always be considered by your doctor.

Muscle diseases

This is another important category of conditions that understandably can go hand-in-hand with fatigue. Unfortunately it includes a number of rare and unusual muscle conditions which can produce easy or early fatiguing of muscles.

Inflammation of muscles

There are a number of conditions that cause muscle weakness and fatigue usually with considerable muscle tenderness. A fever, weight loss and general ill-health are common accompaniments. Blood tests that measure inflammation or muscle damage usually detect such conditions. Elderly people are prone to a condition called polymyalgia rheumatica which responds well to a small dose of steroid drugs. Myositis – simply severely inflamed muscles – which can occur at any age, is rare, but may be caused by viral infection.

Muscle wasting diseases – muscular dystrophies

There are several types of muscle wasting diseases. Most affect children but some may not be evident until the age of thirty or forty years. Muscle weakness with thinning of the shoulder, hand or facial muscles may be the earliest indication of the problem. Sometimes muscles become stiff and it becomes difficult to relax them. If muscle weakness is present and if other members of your family are troubled by similar symptoms it would be advisable to have a checkup with your doctor.

Metabolic muscle diseases

In recent years a variety of rare conditions of a mild or severe nature have been described that produce a disturbance of the muscles' metabolism of fats or carbohydrate which are their main source of energy. These diseases can manifest themselves in young or middle-aged people, sometimes with other members of the family being affected too. Episodes of fatigue, muscle weakness, pain or cramps lasting for hours or days which are brought on by exercise, fasting, exposure to cold or drinking alcohol should make one suspicious. It is now appreciated that such conditions have gone unrecognised until sophisticated diagnostic tests became available over the last ten to twenty years. Assessment of blood levels of lactic acid (a chemical which is the by product of energy production in the muscles), potassium or sodium before and after exercise may be useful and there are a variety of other very specialised tests. Initially it may be difficult to distinguish between mild forms of these conditions and true post-viral fatigue. Specialist assessment is essential and it is worth bearing in mind that some people respond to treatment with vitamin B or with drugs which alter muscle metabolism.

Disturbance in muscle metabolism can also occur in people who drink large quantities of alcohol; from lack of vitamins D, B1 (thiamin) and the minerals potassium and magnesium; and as a side-effect of drugs. The drug groups that cause these side-effects include antibiotics and beta blockers (a drug used for high blood pressure and heart disease). These can all be a cause of muscle weakness and fatigue, so if you have been taking these drugs, perhaps you should have them checked.

Myasthenia gravis

This Latin-derived term simply means 'severe muscle weakness'. Like all the other muscle diseases, it too is rare, but important. It characteristically affects adults but can also occur in children or elderly patients causing profound muscle weakness which is most evident toward the end of the day or after even brief exercise. The muscles are very easily fatigued but not painful and improve quickly with rest. There is no muscle wasting. Drooping eyelids is an early symptom and difficulty chewing or swallowing and double vision may occur in more severe cases. Symptoms may be present for months or years and can be very variable in their severity. Drug treatment is usually very successful.

Case History

Hector Smith

Hector hobbled into the consulting room escorted by his mother. A highly intelligent twenty-nine-year-old computer software expert, he had little time to be troubled by his ills. He greeted me with, 'I've got ME, there is nothing that can be done about it.' At first it seemed a reasonable diagnosis as his muscle fatigue had come on gradually over the previous three years following his fair share of coughs and colds. There had been no acute precipitating infective or other illness. He commented that his muscle fatigue was worse at the end of the day, but there were no aches and pains and he tried to make light of his symptoms.

Examination showed that he had profound muscle weakness in both the arms and legs, which is not a feature of ME. Almost certainly there was an underlying muscle disease and he required urgent referral to a neurologist. After a little reluctance on his part, he saw a neurologist who diagnosed myasthenia gravis – a serious but rare muscle disease. It had progressed to affect almost all the muscles of his body. Fortunately, he responded very well to drug treatment.

This was an all-too-good example of the dangers of making a self-diagnosis of ME (myalgic encephalomyelitis). Anyone with significant fatigue should always see their doctor as there are so many diseases – all requiring different treatment – that could be causing the fatigue *other than* ME.

Diseases of the nervous system

These are usually easier to diagnose than muscle disease because there are relatively few neurological conditions that produce either muscle pain or fatigue. Usually there are other more prominent and distinguishing symptoms. Most will also cause one or more of the following:

- Numbness or tingling especially in the hands or feet.
- Loss of balance or unsteadiness.
- Disturbance in either bowel or bladder function.
- Difficulty in swallowing or with speech.
- Muscle cramps or weakness that is localised to one group of muscles, for example in an arm or leg.
- Muscle wasting.
- Muscle tremors or small jerks.
- Disturbance of vision.

Fatigue and one or some of the above problems may also indicate multiple sclerosis and other degenerative diseases of the nervous system. Anyone with this pattern of symptoms should be assessed by their doctor and a neurologist.

Drug side-effects and toxins

Sometimes fatigue can be a side-effect of an environmental toxin, drug or alcohol. Probably the most common and relevant is alcohol.

Alcohol

The consumption of alcohol, our favourite social poison, has been rising steadily over the last fifty years. The damaging effects of excess alcohol are now well known with the agreed general recommendation that it is unwise to consume more than three units per day for men and one to two units per day for women. A unit is one glass of wine (one-sixth of a 70 cl bottle), a pub measure of spirit, a small glass of sherry or vermouth or half a pint (280 millilitres) of normal strength beer. Home measures of spirits are usually two or three units!

People who consume eight or more units a day run a risk of damage to the liver but this only affects about 10 per cent of heavy drinkers. The other 90 per cent do not escape as there is also an increased risk of heart disease, high blood pressure, stroke, brain damage, nerve damage, stomach ulcers, pancreatic disease, muscle damage, obesity and nutritional deficiencies. The latter combined with the disturbance that alcohol causes to the metabolism is probably the cause of the fatigue that can arise. If you regularly consume between four and seven units of alcohol per day you also run an intermediate risk of these problems.

Very often people with post-infective fatigue or other

fatigue states have learnt to avoid or greatly limit their intake of alcohol and if they haven't then they should.

Case History

Harold Robbs

Harold Robbs was a semi-retired sixty-three-year-old stockbroker. He had had an exciting and dynamic business life. His only complaint was short periods of exhaustion which had been present for many years. A few questions quickly gave me an idea of the cause of the problem. He smoked forty cigarettes a day, had nothing or two cups of tea for breakfast, nothing or a bowl of soup for lunch, and a good meal in the evening, but usually with few vegetables. This was washed down with $1\frac{1}{2}$ litres of wine (twelve units per day).

This he did every day – day in, day out, week in, week out, year in, year out. He said he never felt drunk and never had a hangover. He was clearly someone with a robust constitution. Even so, his blood pressure was increased at 180/100 (the normal range for men is up to 140/90), and blood tests revealed multiple nutritional deficiencies as a result of his poor diet and excessive alcohol intake. Vitamin B1 (thiamin) especially was low enough to affect energy metabolism and cause semi-permanent nerve and brain cell damage.

I advised him to at least halve his cigarette and alcohol consumption, improve his diet and to take some strong multivitamin supplements.

Unfortunately, the success rate of treating such determined characters is low unless they really make the decision to seek help and follow the advice given. Even a modest consumption of alcohol at more than three or four units per day may be enough in some susceptible individuals to affect levels of essential nutrients and to lower energy levels.

Environmental toxins

This is listed by experts as a possible cause of fatigue that should be considered. Relevant toxins include lead, cadmium, possibly mercury, pesticides and organic, usually industrial, chemicals.

There are really two types of exposure to consider. The first is the now 'normal' background exposure to these and other agents that we are all subjected to. At the time of writing there is no good evidence that this background exposure is a distinct cause of fatigue though it may have an influence on child development in the case of lead and cancer risk in the case of many other chemicals.

Cases of distinct mild or severe poisoning do, however, occur in occupational or accidental exposure. If you have had excessive exposure you may well have some knowledge or suspicion of it. Questions about your work, hobbies, and present and past places of living may be relevant factors to discuss with your doctor.

Drugs

Both illicit and medical drugs can produce fatigue. Usage of many illicit drugs including marijuana (pot), cocaine, amphetamines and other stimulants, heroin and its related compounds and hallucinogenic agents such as LSD can produce a wide variety of psychiatric problems that might occasionally be confused with fatigue. A few relevant questions and observations should help to determine if this is a problem.

A more difficult situation is when fatigue is a side-effect of a medically prescribed drug. This can happen with the chronic administration of sedative and tranquillising drugs; drugs for high blood pressure and heart disease called beta blockers (of which there are several types); and occasionally with some antibiotics and other drugs.

The drug is implicated when it appears that the fatigue began after the drugs were first taken. Only careful cessation of the drug under medical supervision will determine if this is the case or not.

Diuretics which promote the loss of water as urine from the body can induce a depletion in the minerals potassium, magnesium and sometimes sodium. This will depend on the type of drug, your age and health, and the type of diet you follow as well as other factors. Measurement of these minerals in the blood which should be performed in the majority of patients with chronic fatigue will easily detect this problem.

Chronic usage of sedative drugs such as diazepam and lorazepam, often used in the treatment of anxiety, can produce a variety of mental symptoms including depression. Withdrawal of these and related benzodiazepine drugs can, according to the manufacturers, result in anxiety, depression, headache, insomnia and physical symptoms, a picture that might be confused with chronic fatigue.

Summary

There is just no substitute for thoroughness and vigilance on the part of those medical practitioners, family doctors, physicians or psychiatrists who care for people with fatigue because there are so many possible causes. For this reason

I have had to go into detail about many conditions which I know has been hard going for the lay person.

If you have symptoms or other features that seem relevant to any of the conditions mentioned, and if you have not already mentioned them to your doctor or specialist, then you should. As you can see with all these possible physical causes for fatigue he or she could do with a little help!

6

Fatigue and nutrition

This is a very important and contentious area. Medical opinion has been divided about the relationship between nutrition and fatigue for over twenty-five years and more recent findings have only fuelled rather than settled the controversy. To better understand what follows it may be useful to first give a little background to the subject of nutrition.

In the past few years, expert national and government committees such as NACNE (National Advisory Committee on Nutritional Education) and COMA (Committee on Medical Aspects of Food) in the UK have been advising us how we, the average citizen, should eat.

Opinion abounds, not just from these and other august bodies, but from individual doctors, nutritionists, health advisors, and alternative and complementary practitioners. In the end, it is easy to be confused by the plethora of advice that bombards the individual. Our own dietary and food choices are influenced, not just by these wise words, but by our likes and dislikes, by our income, upbringing, education and social circumstances. Nutrition and diet, like sex, politics and religion, is a subject on which everyone is an 'expert' and has an opinion even if it is not expressed.

The consensus of opinion, certainly from orthodox committees, is that by and large much of the UK population would be well advised to make certain dietary changes. These include reducing the intakes of sugar (sucrose), salt, animal (i.e. saturated) fats and alcohol, if excessive, and increasing the intakes of fruit, vegetables and more nutritious foods. These changes, it is felt, would help to reduce the incidence of heart disease, high blood pressure, possibly cancer, dental decay and other common health problems. In truth, at best these measures would not completely prevent all these conditions from occurring, but would either reduce the rate at which they show, or delay the age at which they develop. Worthy goals indeed. Much of this advice is good old common sense about healthy eating.

Opinion is, however, quite divided about another aspect of nutrition – the appropriateness of taking vitamin and mineral supplements. Orthodox committees argue that virtually no one needs to take nutritional supplements. In the United Kingdom, as has been shown, supplements are taken by those who usually have the best diets, which may be due both to their concern about health and a willingness to spend money on making sure that they have adequate nutrition.

The information experts use to make their assertions about the nutritional state of the general population comes from a number of surveys conducted in the United Kingdom over the last ten years. Healthy well-fed adults rarely have any major nutritional problems. It is a different situation with children, the elderly and those, of all ages, who are unwell – and this applies to people with fatigue severe enough to disrupt daily life.

A particularly good and relevant example in the United Kingdom is that some 4 per cent of the normal female population of child-bearing age are anaemic – mainly due to a lack of iron as a result of losses due to menstruation. A further 10 per cent may have borderline iron levels. Accordingly, some 10 per cent or more of such women will have a need for iron which cannot be satisfied by their diet and will need to take a supplement on a regular or occasional basis. Iron, as you will see later, is an essential nutrient, deficiency of which can cause mild fatigue.

So much for an introduction! Let's take a look at what individual nutrients do and why they are important to health, fatigue and resistance to infection.

NUTRITION AND METABOLISM

The body is a machine. A very clever one, but like all machines it needs an energy supply and like many machines it has a tendency at times to go wrong. Some of us are lucky to have a Rolls-Royce metabolism, others have one like an old banger. Fortunately, though all bodies can fail to work properly in times of illness, the body's own natural powers of recovery are tremendous and it takes a lot to really disturb the body's metabolism and health. In fact, because of the body's natural robustness and complex metabolism, even a modest nutritional deficiency can be tolerated without much ill-health. However, when several factors combine to suppress health, then problems appear.

As well as the quality and nutritional balance of the diet, factors such as active or recent infection, underlying illness, allergies, general physical fitness and stress can combine together to produce physical problems. For example, the immune system, which helps the body to fight infection, is known to be influenced by nutrition, hormones, stress, presence of infection and allergies – and that is just one of many functions in the body.

There are certain parts of our diet that are essential for good health. They are:

- Energy – mainly from fats and carbohydrates.
- Protein – which provides amino acids essential for health.
- Vitamins.
- Minerals.
- Essential fatty acids – derived from vegetable produce and fish.

Their effects on energy level, mood and resistance to infection is summarised overleaf. The table also indicates how common deficiencies are in average diets in Western countries.

A varied, healthy diet composed mainly of nutritious foods should usually provide these elements in adequate amounts unless there are special requirements or particular health problems. Deficiency of one or more of these essential dietary components results in ill-health. For our purposes it is useful to see what effect these individual nutrients have upon energy level, mood and resistance to infection.

Of course some of these essential nutrients are more important than others in relation to fatigue. Consequently their are individual chapters on iron, magnesium and the B group of vitamins. The other nutrients are covered in a separate chapter.

Effect of Nutrient Deficiencies on Health

Nutrient	Fatigue	Mood	Resistance to infection	Likelihood of deficiency
Protein	YES	YES	YES	RARE
Fats	YES	NO	NO	RARE
Carbohydrates	YES	NO	NO	RARE
Essential fatty acids	POSSIBLY	NO	YES	RARE

Vitamins

A	NO	NO	YES	VERY RARE
B Complex	YES	YES	YES	COMMON
C	YES	YES	YES	RARE
D	NO	NO	NO	VERY RARE
E	NO	NO	SLIGHT	VERY RARE
K	NO	NO	NO	VERY RARE

Minerals

Iron	YES	YES	YES	COMMON
Calcium	NO	NO	NO	COMMON IN ELDERLY
Potassium	YES	NO	NO	RARE
Magnesium	YES	YES	NO	UNCERTAIN
Zinc	NO	YES	YES	UNCERTAIN
Other trace elements	NO	NO	SLIGHT	VERY RARE

Fatigue and iron

Iron deficiency is considered by most nutritionists to be the commonest deficiency worldwide resulting in anaemia and a host of other health problems including fatigue.

Iron is one of the essential nutrients known as 'trace elements'. It is perhaps the best known of those essential trace elements that are required in tiny amounts to perform specific functions relating to health.

Lack of iron has long been linked with fatigue. Indeed the first reports of this can be traced back to the sixteenth century when Dr Johannes Lange, a German physician, wrote of the condition then termed 'chlorosis'. This he described in his classic paper entitled *Concerning the Disease of the Virgins* which was published in 1554. In this paper, Dr Lange describes a young woman, Anno, who 'is desired in marriage by many suitors, of great excellency and illustrious birth' whom her father is compelled to refuse 'because of the weakness of his daughter'. She also complains that her once rosy complexion has become pale, that she easily develops shortness of breath when dancing or climbing the stairs and that her stomach loathes food, particularly meat – a rich source of iron. This condition was termed 'chlorosis' because the very pale complexion took on a faint green tinge!

Subsequently anaemia (a lack of the oxygen carrying haemoglobin) due to iron deficiency was determined to be the cause of this condition called chlorosis – a troublesome cause of fatigue of virgins in years gone by! Such extreme cases are rarely seen these days in developed countries. However, mild or moderate iron deficiency is, as we shall see, quite common and is a significant cause of fatigue and other health problems, particularly in menstruating women who have a low intake of iron from their diet.

IRON – WHAT IT DOES

Iron is needed for the production of the blood pigment haemoglobin which carries oxygen around the body and colours the blood red. A lack of iron leads to a fall in the level of haemoglobin and as a result a fall in the amount of oxygen reaching the tissues. This may not be very noticeable when you are at rest but even just walking up stairs requires extra production of energy which in turn will need an additional amount of oxygen. If the oxygen carrying capacity of the blood is reduced then the muscles will not receive the additional oxygen they require, and we will have reduced work capacity as a result of the anaemia.

This can also occur in mild iron deficiency without a fall in the level of haemoglobin. Iron is needed for another oxygen carrying compound called myoglobin which is found in muscles and which may not function adequately in deficiency conditions.

Finally iron is needed for the function of some enzymes (complex proteins that direct the chemical reactions of the body) that influence growth, resistance to infection and nervous system function.

WHO'S LACKING IRON?

You might justifiably imagine that, as iron deficiency was first described four to five centuries ago, medical science would have nearly eradicated this problem. Far from it. Iron deficiency is alive and well in all communities, rich and poor, in the latter half of the twentieth century.

A recent detailed survey of the nutritional state of the adult population (age eighteen to sixty-four years) was conducted in the UK by the Department of Health and the Ministry of Agriculture, Fisheries and Food. The results were published as a book, the size of a small telephone directory, *The Dietary and Nutritional Survey of British Adults*. From it we can discover just how common deficiency of iron and many other nutrients are in the UK. Great care was taken by the authors of this important survey to assess over 2,000 adults who were living in all the main regions of the United Kingdom and represented all the main social groups including the unemployed. It also included those who were unwell and asked if they were eating properly or not and those who were dieting. The survey is therefore considered to be representative of the whole population of the United Kingdom.

The findings of the survey in relation to iron deficiency were particularly revealing and showed that many of us are not as healthy as we should be. A total of 4 per cent of all women aged between eighteen and sixty-four years were anaemic – having a reduced concentration of the oxygen carrying pigment haemoglobin in the blood. This was considered to be mainly due to a lack of iron. Other blood changes supported this conclusion. Only 1 per cent of men were anaemic with a low haemoglobin.

So we could expect that some 4 per cent of adult women might feel tired or have other health problems as a result of being anaemic. That was not the end of it as the study rightly included a very sensitive test that gives a measure of the reserves of iron stored in the body. This test is called the serum ferritin which over the last decade or so has begun to be widely regarded as the best way to accurately assess iron state. The level of ferritin (which is a protein in the blood that carries iron around) will fall before the level of haemoglobin has dropped. A low level of ferritin will mean that there are reduced levels of iron in the bone marrow and possibly tissues such as the brain, muscles, skin, hair and nails. A low ferritin level in someone with a haemo-globin level that is normal can be associated with a variety of symptoms including mild fatigue.

A total of 14 per cent of all women in this survey had ferritin levels below a serum value of 13 micrograms per litre, considered to be the lower end of normal. This rose to 21 per cent in the thirty-five to forty-nine year age group falling to 5 per cent in the fifty to sixty-four year age group, undoubtedly due to the menopause, which despite its own problems does mean the end of periods and a decrease in the body's demand for iron.

The increased risk of iron deficiency described may quite seriously lie behind the still widely held opinion that women, particularly those of child-bearing age, are the weaker and fairer (paler) sex. Perhaps you might think that the United Kingdom is an exception? Well, a number of detailed studies in the normal population and in blood from a variety of developed countries shows much the same picture.

In 1976, a survey of the iron status of 1,105 Canadians by Dr Leslie Valberg and colleagues from the University of Western Ontario concluded that the iron stores were greatly reduced in approximately 25 per cent of children, 30 per cent of adolescents, 30 per cent of menstruating

women, 60 per cent of pregnant women and 3 per cent of
men. Only 2 per cent of the total group surveyed, however,
were actually anaemic.

A more recent survey performed in the United States of
America, which was the equivalent of the UK survey, was
published in 1986. This survey was termed the National
Health and Nutritional Examination Survey (NHANES II)
and was a survey of 2,829 individuals between the ages
eighteen and sixty-four years. From this survey it was
estimated that only 0.2 per cent of adult men were anaemic
but 2.6 per cent of women aged eighteen and forty-four
years and 1.9 per cent of women aged forty-five and sixty-
four years were anaemic.

Further blood examinations and calculations of the
percentage of these groups who had low stores of iron,
with or without anaemia, gave estimates of 1.8 per cent of
men, 22.3 per cent of women aged eighteen to forty-four
years and 7.6 per cent of women aged forty-five to sixty-
four years.

THE IMPORTANCE OF IRON DEFICIENCY

Years ago it was thought that iron deficiency anaemia did
not produce symptoms until the level of haemoglobin fell
to a value of 10 grams in the blood. In fact in more recent
years a whole host of minor symptoms have been shown to
be related to iron deficiency with either a slightly reduced
or even low-normal haemoglobin.

These minor problems include:

- Recurrent mouth ulceration.
- A sore or burning tongue or mouth.
- Cracking at the corners of the mouth.
- Excessive scalp hair loss in women.

- Split or brittle nails which may become flattened.
- Poor appetite or in children a desire to eat dirt, paint or other unpalatable things.
- Mild digestive problems especially in children.
- Occasionally difficulty in swallowing.
- Possibly craving for ice or cold drinks.
- Reduced resistance to infection especially with candida (thrush).
- Poor temperature regulation.
- Poor concentration.
- Reduced classroom performance in children.
- FATIGUE.

It must be pointed out that all of these complaints can each have a wide variety of other causes even if you have several of them. Thus there is no substitute for a proper medical and nutritional assessment of your symptoms.

Case History

Rosie O'Grady

Though only twenty-eight, Rosie had four children. She and her husband had always planned to have a large family. However, since the birth of her last child six months previously, she had developed increasing fatigue. Her diet had been excellent, and her pregnancies uncomplicated with a good weight gain and no anaemia. Even so, she felt very run down. Coping with four children and breastfeeding was no small task. Indeed, she had either been pregnant or breastfeeding for sixty-five of the preceding eighty-eight months!

Her blood tests had shown that she had a borderline

haemoglobin, 11.7 grams (the normal range being 11.5–16.5). Serum ferritin (a sensitive test of iron reserves) was low.

I suggested a strong iron supplement and multivitamin supplement, and that she continued with her excellent diet. Her energy level gradually improved over the next six months, when she became pregnant again!

Pregnancy and breastfeeding can impose considerable strain on the body. Iron requirements may increase or remain the same depending upon the person's diet and physiology. It is advisable to space pregnancies some eighteen months or more apart to give your body a chance to recover full health.

STUDIES ON IRON DEFICIENCY AND FATIGUE

Much of the medical research that has brought us this full understanding of the picture of iron deficiency has taken place in the last fifteen years but the first properly conducted work on iron and fatigue was published as long ago as 1960!

In 1960, Dr Ernest Beutler and colleagues from Chicago decided to study a group of chronically fatigued women giving them each iron tablets and placebo (dummy) tablets and see what the effect would be. They had got the idea from some German researchers who, during the 1940s and 1950s, had suggested that there was indeed a connection between mild iron deficiency and fatigue.

The group of subjects who volunteered were all women from the out-patients departments of the University of Chicago Clinics or were students at the University of Chicago. They all complained of fatigue with or without other symptoms such as headaches, dizziness and nervousness.

They all had to have a thorough physical examination, which was normal, and not be anaemic – with a haemoglobin level of 12 grams or more. In other words they all had to fall into the category of 'fatigued but nothing physically wrong with you'.

Next they underwent a series of further tests to assess their iron state. This included having a number of blood tests and a bone marrow sample taken as, in 1960, serum ferritin measurements were not available. They were then categorised into one of two groups depending upon the level of their iron stores. After further assessment of their symptoms they were then all started on the treatment phase of the study receiving either iron tablets or the placebo for three months, followed by a break for one month, then a further three months of the placebo or iron. In this way every woman received both iron and placebo so a comparison could be made between the two treatments.

Dr Beutler and his colleagues also took care to make sure that the women did not know which treatment they were receiving at which time and that the doctors seeing the women or performing the tests did so without knowing who was receiving which treatment. Thus both the women and the doctors were 'blind' to the treatment they were being given. This was in fact one of the first ever carefully designed trials and the publication title, *Iron therapy in chronically fatigued non-anaemic women: a double-blind study*, reflects this.

A total of twenty-nine women completed the study, each receiving placebo for three months and iron as 300 milligrams of ferrous sulphate three times daily for three months. This is a very substantial dose of iron and one that would certainly raise iron levels significantly. Indeed during the study those with the lowest levels of iron experienced a rise in haemoglobin of nearly 0.5 of a gram when receiving iron and either no change or a small fall in haemoglobin when receiving placebo.

These twenty-nine women were analysed by dividing them into two groups; those who had definite evidence of low iron stores (twenty-two women) and those whose iron stores appeared to be normal (seven women). Each was asked to decide whether they felt less fatigued on the iron tablets or on the placebo or if there was no preference. If the iron was no different from placebo then we would expect that there would be approximately equal numbers of women preferring iron and placebo. This was not the case.

In the group of twenty-two women with low iron levels at the start of the study fifteen had a preference for iron, five for placebo and two had no particular preference. In the group of seven women with satisfactory iron stores at the start two had a preference for iron and five for placebo. A statistical analysis of these results showed that preference for iron in the iron-deficient group would have been most unlikely to occur by chance. So the preference for iron was likely to be due to a true beneficial effect of iron itself and not anything else.

There was therefore some modest benefit to giving iron supplements to chronically fatigued women who were not anaemic but who had evidence of low iron stores. It is highly likely that the levels of iron in the muscles and other tissues increased during iron therapy though this was not actually measured.

We can also conclude that treatment with iron is not a cure-all for fatigue, being more likely to benefit those who are deficient, even if only mildly, than those who are not.

Despite the care taken by the authors, their work is open to some criticism. The number of women in the trial was small and the assessment of the treatment's effectiveness relied upon the women's own perception of how they felt rather than upon some independent method. Also the dosage of iron was very high, some two to three times the amount that is now usually given in the treatment of iron deficiency. These high doses can cause side-effects of indigestion, diarrhoea, constipation or give a dark colour to the stool. This last possibility may have enabled some of the women to ascertain whether they were taking the iron or the placebo, and this in turn could have influenced their responses to the doctors' questions about the progress. To minimise this effect the dummy or placebo tablets also contained a substance, bismuth subcarbonate, which also darkened the stools.

Since this study, there has been surprisingly little work on fatigue and iron. In 1966 a survey of 165 women and 130 men all aged fifteen years or over was conducted in the United Kingdom by Drs Wood and Elwood. They were looking at the prevalence of anaemia and whether this was related to fatigue or not. Three of the 130 men were found to be anaemic and fifteen of the 165 women were anaemic. Despite this these doctors did not find any association between the patients' self-assessment of fatigue and the concentration of haemoglobin in either the men or the women. There was some small indication that those with a low level of haemoglobin were likely to feel more fatigued. However, the number of women in this last category was small, only eight, and the authors rightly concluded that, 'More evidence is required from a larger sample of severely iron-deficient subjects'. Drs Wood and Elwood did find, however, that a pale appearance was associated with an increased risk of anaemia.

Since the 1960s there have been a considerable number of studies looking more closely at the effects of iron deficiency and anaemia on health but these have mainly

been in young children and not in adults. In brief, these
have shown that correction of iron-deficient anaemia can
result in improved weight gain, accelerated development
and better concentration and performance in the classroom. Poor mental performance has been observed in
children who are iron deficient but not actually anaemic
and this may improve after iron supplements are taken.

There is thus increasing evidence that both actual anaemia and mild iron deficiency without anaemia are quite
common in women of child-bearing age and in boys and
girls especially of pre-school age, with the result that both
their physical and mental capabilities may be reduced. Such
individuals may go to their doctor complaining of mild
fatigue, and their complaints should be taken seriously;
and as an editorial in the leading medical journal the
Lancet, said, '. . . it is well worth estimating the serum-iron
level and the saturation of the iron binding capacity [now
superseded by the serum ferritin] in women of all ages and
in patients over the age of 60 with persistent fatigue, that
does not respond to treatment of their primary condition,
even when there is no evidence of overt iron-deficiency
anaemia.' It was good advice when it appeared in 1968 and
it still is now.

HOW CAN I TELL IF I AM LACKING IN IRON?

The short answer is you will have to go to your doctor for
a blood test measuring both the level of haemoglobin and
the serum ferritin. If this latter test is not available then the
measurement of the serum iron and the iron binding
capacity will give much the same information. However, a
little care should be taken if the serum iron is measured. It
is better not to have eaten for four or more hours before the

blood sample is taken because the level of iron can go up after a meal. It can also fall significantly from four days before the start of a period to the end.

It is easy to say that everyone should have these tests performed. In practice some assessment of the likelihood of iron deficiency needs to be made before undertaking blood tests and this may give some clue as to the possible cause if deficiency is indeed found.

Risk factors for iron deficiency

Poor intake   This results from a diet low in iron-rich foods e.g. meat, fortified breakfast cereals and protein-rich vegetarian foods – beans, nuts, seeds and eggs.

Poor absorption   This is due to dietary factors and is found most likely in full or semi-vegetarians. A relatively low intake of vitamin C from fresh fruit and vegetables and consuming tea – a good source of tannin – or unleavened grain products such as bran or chapatis, which are rich in phytic acid, will result in a significant fall in the amount of iron that is absorbed into the body from a vegetarian meal.

Poor absorption is also due to digestive factors affecting either the stomach, the small bowel or the pancreas; e.g. after operations removing all or part of the stomach, coeliac disease and other serious bowel disorders.

Increased demand   In rapidly growing children, during pregnancy and breastfeeding but usually only when intakes are also poor or borderline.

Increased losses   From menstruation because of heavy, prolonged or frequent periods. Blood loss may also occur from the gut because of internal bleeding due to a peptic ulcer, drug usage including aspirin, anti-arthritis drugs and steroids, cancer of the stomach or colon, inflammation of the bowel as in colitis or Crohn's disease and from intolerance to cow's milk in children.

So you can see that there are a potentially large number of risk factors to be considered. A not infrequent situation is a woman in her thirties or forties who is having heavier periods, and who over the last few years had changed her diet by reducing her intake of meat, a good source of iron, but is still consuming some tea and bran that can reduce the percentage of iron that is absorbed. She certainly has some of the risk factors for iron deficiency and one would be even more suspicious if she also had recurrent mouth ulcers, tongue soreness or cracking at the corners of her mouth as well as fatigue.

WHAT SHOULD HAPPEN IF YOU ARE IRON DEFICIENT?

If tests have shown that you are anaemic then your doctor may need to perform a number of other tests to determine whether the anaemia is due to a lack of iron or possibly due to a lack of vitamin B12 (folic acid) or due to some other condition.

The cause of the iron deficiency will need to be determined which will mean making some assessment of your dietary intake, finding out whether you have digestive problems or are losing small amounts of blood from bleeding internally, or are losing excessive amounts of blood with your monthly period. A physical and, if appropriate, gynaecological examination are usually needed and if the cause is uncertain some tests to look at blood loss from the bowel. The latter is particularly important in men over the age of forty and women over the age of fifty when the risk of a growth in the bowel increases. Sometimes no further tests would be necessary as, for example, in the case of a student in her early twenties, who is not eating a very good diet, has been having slightly heavy periods and is otherwise well. A course of iron for three to six months with a repeat of her blood tests to make sure that her anaemia has been corrected is probably all that is required.

INCREASING THE IRON IN THE DIET

This is the most important part of treating iron deficiency. On average, children aged between seven and ten need 6.7 milligrams of iron per day; adult women who are menstruating need 11.4 milligrams and men and non-menstruating women need 6.7 milligrams. Intakes lower than this may be enough for some people. It is possible to obtain about twice these levels from a healthy diet. The foods with the highest content of iron are: red meat, whole wheat and cereals, eggs, shell fish (cockles in particular), nuts (particularly almonds), beans, green vegetables, and dried fruit. Here is a list of 100 grams (4 oz) portions of foods containing iron:

Iron-rich foods

	milligrams per 100 grams (4 oz) of food
Cereals	
Wheat bran (but not well-absorbed)	12.9
Rice	0.5

Meat
Beef (lean, cooked)   1.4
Rump steak (boneless sirloin, lean only, grilled)   3.5
Lamb (lean, roast)   2.5
Lamb kidney   12.0
Pork (lean, grilled)   1.2
Pig liver (stewed)   17.0
Chicken (dark meat)   1.0
Chicken (liver, fried)   9.1

Eggs
Eggs, whole (boiled)   2.0
Egg yolk (raw)   6.1

Fish
Sardines (canned in oil)   2.9
Trout (steamed)   1.0
Crab (boiled)   1.3
Prawns or shrimps (boiled)   1.1
Mussels (boiled)   7.7
Oysters (raw)   6.0
Scallops (steamed)   3.0

Nuts
Almonds   4.2
Brazils   2.8
Coconut (fresh)   2.1

Dairy
Cheddar cheese   0.4

Vegetables and pulses
Haricot beans (boiled)   2.5
Mung beans (raw)   8.0

Red kidney beans	6.7
Avocado pear	1.5
Lentils (boiled)	2.4
Butter (lima) beans (boiled)	1.7
Parsley	8.0
Spring greens – cabbage (boiled)	1.3
Leeks	2.0

Fruit

Apricots	0.4
Bananas	0.4
Blackberries	0.9
Dates (dried)	1.6
Figs (dried)	4.2
Sultanas or golden raisins (dried)	1.8
Strawberries	0.7

As well as eating plenty of iron-rich foods you can easily increase the amount of iron that is absorbed by your body by eating foods containing vitamin C, like fruit and vegetables. Normally only 10 per cent of the iron in the food we eat is actually absorbed into the body, and the rest just passes through with the waste matter. When you are deficient in iron the body adapts to increase the percentage that is absorbed from the diet.

Tannin is a chemical found in tea and is excellent at reducing the amount of iron absorbed by about two thirds! So if you want your cup of tea and you need your iron then keep two hours or more between your meal and your 'cuppa'. This only applies to the iron from non-meat sources so the tea-drinking vegetarian is particularly vulnerable. Equally, if you need to take some iron tablets, don't wash them down with that traditional British beverage. Use a glass of fruit juice instead as its vitamin C content will mean that you get nearly twice as much iron out of it.

TAKING IRON TABLETS

In practice most people with iron deficient anaemia or reduced iron stores will need to take iron tablets for a while. This should be for between three and six months depending on your response to treatment.

Iron tablets may be a necessary evil as they can have side-effects too. Often this is just a darkening of the stools due to the unabsorbed iron, but they can also cause constipation, diarrhoea or abdominal discomfort. When this happens it is best to reduce the dose, taking smaller amounts at any one time, and take the tablets with meals that include fruit or vegetables. Very occasionally it is necessary to try a variety of different iron preparations before finding one that is suitable. Sometimes iron needs to be given by injection.

CAN I JUST GO AND TAKE SOME IRON ANYWAY?

A lot of people do take iron tablets or multivitamins with iron on a regular or occasional basis without seeking any medical advice. This is unlikely to be harmful if the dose is small, in the region of 10 to 15 milligrams per day, close to an average dietary intake. In fact it is estimated that some 10 per cent of menstruating women should be taking this amount of iron to make up for their monthly losses which could only be provided by a very nutritious and expensive diet.

It would also be appropriate for quite a substantial proportion of young children between the ages of a year and five years to be taking modest amounts of iron, perhaps combined with vitamins. This might also apply to older girls at the onset of puberty especially if a good intake of iron from the diet cannot be guaranteed. Healthy men and boys in their teens are unlikely to need iron supplements.

Taking large amounts of iron or taking iron for long periods of time without checking with your doctor can be dangerous. A high as opposed to a low level of iron in the blood is now thought to be a risk factor for heart disease and this is relevant to men and women who have ceased menstruating. There are also a few individuals whose bodies are too efficient at absorbing iron. This condition is called haemochromatosis and occurs in about 1 per cent of the normal population. It runs in families so anyone with a relative with this condition should not take iron tablets without checking with their doctor.

So, too much or too little iron can affect your health. Nature likes a balance and in the case of iron it's a fine balance. The evidence shows that iron deficiency is a common finding in both developed and developing countries and a potentially important and under-diagnosed cause of fatigue in the general population.

8

Fatigue and magnesium

Many of you reading this book will have heard about the use of magnesium in chronic fatigue. Perhaps you have quickly turned to this chapter to see what it says and whether there is anything new.

Well, I have no new breakthroughs or revelations to report but I would like to put the issue of magnesium in perspective and give some hopefully useful information about ways you and your doctor can improve the balance of this and other essential nutrients in your body. But first some background.

In 1991, three doctors in Southampton, England, conducted a study that looked at the magnesium balance and effect of magnesium, given by injection, to a group of patients with chronic fatigue. The results of that study which were published in the medical journal the *Lancet* received substantial publicity on television, radio and in national and provincial newspapers in the United Kingdom. Sufferers and journalists alike were hungry for just this type of news and greeted the 80 per cent success rate with enthusiasm.

The merits and limitations of this study will be considered later but one important lesson is that a large majority of people are looking for a simple one-shot cure when it is extremely unlikely that this will be the case for the majority of people suffering with chronic fatigue. This book is broken up into chapters dealing with individual nutrients and types of conditions for simplicity, and not because I am trying to say that one approach is better than another. That is not the case. There are merits in many of the approaches discussed in the book and it very much depends on which approach suits you and your symptoms at the end of the day.

MAGNESIUM – WHAT IT DOES

Magnesium is mainly found in muscles, bones and nerves. It helps maintain the electrical balance in these tissues, and is also involved as a helping factor in energy-forming chemical reactions. In muscles magnesium is needed for the smooth contraction and relaxation of the muscle fibres. Magnesium balance is influenced by the presence of other minerals, including calcium, sodium and potassium. A lack of magnesium mostly affects nerve and muscle function, and this includes not only the limb and back muscles but also those of the heart, gut and blood vessels.

WHO IS LACKING MAGNESIUM?

Severe deficiency of magnesium is rare and normally only occurs as a result of significant prolonged illness, starvation, severe weight loss, alcoholism, severe digestive problems, and prolonged diarrhoea and vomiting. The bones and muscles act as a good store of magnesium, so it is hard for deficiencies to develop quickly.

Some drugs also increase the loss of magnesium from the body, and this includes types of diuretics – water tablets – called thiazides. These drugs are known to cause loss of potassium too and the elderly seem particularly prone to depletion.

So much for severe deficiency. Mild deficiency may cause some problems too. The issue has been raised in recent years that mild magnesium depletion may be found in connection with certain complaints, including fatigue. A mild lack of magnesium may only show up in a lowered red blood cell concentration of magnesium. This has been found both in patients with fatigue and also in women suffering from premenstrual syndrome. There is some overlap between these two conditions, as you will see in Chapter 11. Low red cell values of magnesium do suggest that other tissues, particularly muscles and nerves, may also have reduced concentrations of this mineral, and as a result may be functioning less efficiently.

Magnesium in the average United Kingdom diet is mainly provided by cereals (33 per cent) and green vegetables (18 per cent). Modest amounts are also found in meat and animal products. So eating a wholesome diet should provide you with plenty of magnesium. The *Dietary and Nutritional Survey of British Adults* showed that average intakes for men and women were 323 and 237 milligrams per day respectively, and these values are in excess of the estimated average requirements for men and women. Demand for magnesium, however, increases substantially during pregnancy and breastfeeding, and this is the time when relative magnesium depletion might develop if the quality of your diet is not maintained. Women who have twin pregnancies, a slow or difficult first labour, or who give birth to their second child before seventeen years of age, are particularly at risk of magnesium depletion.

Giving magnesium supplements during pregnancy has been shown to be associated with a slight reduction in the rate of premature babies and fewer complications during pregnancy for the mother and for the newborn infant. As it appears that the demands of pregnancy may only be met by eating a very good diet, certainly fatigue persisting after delivery could in part be due to magnesium (or iron) depletion and this should be borne in mind.

It is also possible that a mild magnesium deficit can occur as a result of a poor quality diet and not just because it has a low magnesium content. For example, the amount of magnesium lost in the urine can be increased by consuming alcohol and having a high dietary intake of glucose and other sugars. The body's overall balance of magnesium appears to be improved by having a nutritious diet with plenty of protein, especially animal protein. Bran and other unleavened wheat products, such as chapatis, may also impede the absorption of magnesium from the diet because of their phytic acid content.

So it is not just how much magnesium you eat but the content of other foods and nutrients in the diet that influences the absorption and balance of this mineral. There is also some suggestion that genetic make-up may have a mild effect on how efficient different people are at retaining magnesium in their body. This type of effect is known to occur with potassium and sodium, and influences the risk of blood pressure problems developing.

In summary, it is hard to develop severe magnesium depletion, but mild depletion could occur as a result of eating a poorly balanced diet, following the increased demands of pregnancy, or as a result of some other predisposing factors. Perhaps a viral or other infection can also disturb the body's metabolism in a way that loosens its grip on this mineral.

THE IMPORTANCE OF MAGNESIUM
DEFICIENCY

Because of magnesium's relationship with other minerals, and the fact that severe deficiency only occurs in people with an illness, it has not been easy to determine exactly what the features of a pure deficiency of this mineral are. Experimental magnesium deficiency has been achieved by Professor M.E. Shils and colleagues at Cornell University Medical College in New York. This was not easy. A low magnesium diet had to be consumed for nearly four months. Anorexia, nausea and apathy occurred frequently, and always occurred before the development of other features. These included personality changes, muscle spasms, tremors and muscle twitches. Changes in calcium and potassium levels were also found to occur. Symptoms of nausea, apathy and minor muscle spasms may thus be the first signs of a mild magnesium lack.

Muscle strength is reduced in alcoholics with a lowered level of magnesium in the serum or water component of the blood. Reduced efficiency of muscle contraction and relaxation has recently been described in a few patients with normal serum magnesium values but with reduced levels in their red blood cells. This work was conducted by Dr John Howard at Biolab Medical Unit in London which also took part in the work on magnesium and fatigue by Dr Cox and colleagues (see below).

Supplements of magnesium may also appear to have a beneficial effect on blood sugar control, and small changes in the levels of magnesium in the blood can accompany recovery from depression (which is often accompanied by fatigue) with a previously low blood magnesium value reverting to normal after drug treatment.

So magnesium seems to have a wide range of effects on

body metabolism in ways that could influence fatigue and mood.

MAGNESIUM IN FATIGUE

During the 1970s and 1980s there was considerable interest in the use of several different magnesium supplements in France in the treatment of a condition known as 'spasmophilia'. This condition is characterised by muscle aches and pains, tingling in the feet and hands, chest discomfort, headache, giddiness and minor mental disturbance. The results of treatment did not, however, appear to convince many researchers outside France.

In the 1980s, as has already been mentioned, a number of doctors observed lowered red cell magnesium values in women with premenstrual syndrome. But it was only in March 1991 that the *Lancet* medical journal carried the report by Drs Cox, Campbell and Dowson, 'Red Blood Cell Magnesium and Chronic Fatigue Syndrome'. This paper was really a report on two studies. In the first, twenty patients with chronic fatigue syndrome had been found to have lowered red blood cell magnesium concentrations when compared with twenty healthy control subjects (matched for age, sex and social class). It appeared the difference was small, as those with fatigue had a magnesium level that was only some 7 per cent lower than the healthy subjects but this difference was statistically significant.

They then went on to test a different group of patients who attended the doctors at the Centre for Study of Complementary Medicine, or who were referred there by their general practitioners. All those in the study had to have been experiencing fatigue that had lasted longer than six months and less than eighteen months.

Approximately two-thirds of the thirty-two subjects recruited for the trial were women, with the average age of all patients being late thirties. Again, they were found to have low red blood cell magnesium levels. They were divided into two groups. One was to receive magnesium sulphate (1 gram in 2 millilitres) by injection, and the other was to receive a placebo, also by injection, each at weekly intervals for six weeks. Neither group knew which of the two injections they were receiving.

Their symptoms were carefully followed with a standard questionnaire. Those who received the magnesium, as compared with those who were given the placebo, reported improvements in energy level, reduced pain and in their emotional reactions. There were no significant changes in the scores for sleep, degree of social isolation or physical mobility. Overall the improvement greatly favoured the magnesium rather than the placebo preparation. At the end of the study, twelve of the fifteen magnesium-treated patients (80 per cent) felt that they had benefited from the treatment, but only three of the seventeen receiving the placebo said that they had felt better. Furthermore, the red cell magnesium levels had returned to normal in all patients receiving the magnesium injection, but in only one patient on the placebo.

The authors concluded that, 'The findings show that magnesium may have a role in chronic fatigue syndrome', and that, 'the results should be viewed with caution'. This latter comment was because the trial was relatively small and had only lasted for six weeks.

The research was funded by the ME Action Campaign in the United Kingdom, and stimulated a great deal of interest. The authors have acknowledged that they are continuing with other trials of magnesium therapy in chronic fatigue states, and the results of this research will be awaited with interest.

Since then the medical journal that published the trial, the *Lancet*, has also carried a number of letters questioning the validity of the results. Dr Clague and colleagues from the Department of Medicine at the University of Liverpool looked at a small group of twelve patients with chronic fatigue, none of whom had evidence of a magnesium deficiency on a series of tests. Not surprisingly, perhaps, none of them reported benefit when given magnesium. So magnesium cannot be regarded as a cure-all.

My own experience is perhaps relevant here. Certainly I have seen some patients with chronic fatigue who have had reduced levels of red cell magnesium as the major abnormal finding. Many, but by no means all, have reported benefit after taking supplements, usually by mouth, for several months. However, I have found it virtually impossible to predict who will do well with this approach. Additionally, I measured the level of red cell magnesium in fifty-eight consecutive adult patients who had not been taking supplements in the preceding four weeks. They were a very mixed group of men and women with a wide variety of both physical and mental complaints, and some of them were troubled by fatigue.

They all completed a detailed questionnaire asking about their physical and mental symptoms. Their answers to the several questions relating to fatigue did not show that those with the lowest red cell magnesiums complained more of fatigue. It is important to remember, however, that this was not a group of patients with chronic fatigue but one with a wide variety of complaints.

Are you confused?

You should be and many doctors certainly are. Essentially it seems that those most likely to benefit from magnesium supplementation are those who have some evidence of a relative deficiency. Those patients who have levels well into the normal range are not expected to benefit and there is a large grey area in the middle.

The real question is to try and identify those with fatigue who are most likely to benefit from magnesium supplements.

Case History

Chris Farmer

Chris's work as a Prison Officer was severely disrupted by repeated throat and chest infections over the course of three or four months. Many of these infections required treatment by antibiotics from his general practitioner. As well as a sore throat or cough, he also experienced fever, generalised aches and pains and also joint pains and stiffness, which were usually present whilst the infection was active.

He never fully recovered from each infection and the chronic fatigue meant he could work only half duties, mainly behind a desk. He appeared to have true ME.

The recent birth of his second child had meant that disturbed nights added to his problems of fatigue. In view of his good diet I was surprised to find that his red cell magnesium level was reduced at 1.8 millimols per litre (the normal range is 2.08–3) and his serum zinc was also reduced at 10 millimols per litre (the normal range is 11.5–20). Taking some extra care with his diet and starting him on multivitamins together with supplements of zinc and magnesium, which his general practitioner was pleased to prescribe, was followed by an improvement over the course of nine months.

The main problem was to make sure he avoided getting further chest or throat infections, and though he had two during the course of this period, neither required antibiotics. As the muscular aches and pains lessened, perhaps because of the magnesium supplements, he increased his level of physical activity very gradually and sensibly. Eventually he was able to either go swimming or jog gently for three miles every day. Although he was fitter than the doctor, he was still a little dissatisfied because he wasn't quite back to where he had been before the illness began.

His levels of magnesium and zinc rose very satisfactorily to the normal range and I suggested that he tail off his supplements but continue with a good diet. Quite why his levels of zinc and magnesium had been low in the first place is not clear, perhaps the original infection had triggered some change in metabolism, but clearly he was in a rut and the supplements, taking care with his diet and gradually increasing his exercise level helped him to come out of it.

HOW CAN I TELL IF I AM LACKING IN MAGNESIUM?

As always, this is an important question, and again this is difficult to answer, particularly as the degree of deficiency described by the Southampton researchers was relatively small. It is not known what percentage of patients complaining of fatigue have low red cell magnesium values, and in what percentage of these the taking of magnesium supplements would really be beneficial. Again it is best to assess those who might be at risk of magnesium depletion, which would include:

- Those on a poor diet, low in green vegetables and cereals.

- Those on a diet low in protein.
- Those with an excessive alcohol consumption.
- Those with chronic diarrhoea or weight loss.
- Those taking thiazide-type diuretics (water tablets).
- Those with symptoms suggestive of mild magnesium deficiency – fatigue, muscle cramps, apathy – without any other obvious cause.

In the end, there is no substitute for assessment by a medical practitioner, including assessment of both serum and red cell magnesium values, which would help to decide the issue. Low levels in serum would be found only rarely, but a reduced red cell value would suggest that it might be appropriate to try a course of magnesium supplements.

TREATING MAGNESIUM DEFICIENCY THROUGH DIET

In theory, it should be easy to raise magnesium levels by eating a good diet, rich in magnesium. As already mentioned, all green vegetables contain lots of magnesium because the green pigment, chlorophyll, requires this mineral to achieve its green colour. Cereals, nuts, seeds, as well as meat products are all good sources of magnesium. A list of the most important foods follows:

Magnesium-rich foods

	milligrams per 100 grams (4 oz) of food
Cereals	
Wheatbran (not well-absorbed)	520
Wholemeal (whole wheat) flour	140

Oatmeal (raw)   110
Porridge oats (cooked)   13
Wholemeal (whole wheat) bread   93
White bread   26
Muesli   100

Meat
Beef (lean, cooked)   11
Lamb (lean, cooked)   12
Chicken meat (roast)   24

Fish
Cod (baked)   26
Herring (grilled)   32
Kipper (baked)   18
Salmon (steamed)   29
Sardines (canned in oil)   52

Nuts
Almonds   260
Brazil   410
Walnuts   130
Peanuts   180

Dairy
Dried skimmed milk   117
Fresh whole milk   12

Vegetables and pulses
Butter (lima) beans (boiled)   33
Haricot beans (boiled)   45
Mung beans (raw)   170
Chick peas (dhal) (cooked)   67
Spinach (boiled)   59

Sweetcorn (boiled)	45
Potatoes (baked with skins)	24
Avocado pear	29
Fruit (raw)	
Pineapple (fresh)	17
Apricots (fresh)	12
Apricots (dried)	65
Bananas	42
Blackberries	30
Dates (dried)	59
Sultanas (golden raisins)	35
Prunes (dried)	27

The average daily requirement of magnesium is 200 milligrams for women and 250 milligrams for men. For children aged between seven and ten years it is 150 milligrams. Intakes less than this may be adequate for some people. Intakes of 50 milligrams more per day for each of these figures would be considered to be very good.

Making the most of magnesium

Other dietary measures may also help you retain the magnesium you ingest:

- Avoid consuming large amounts of foods rich in sugar and glucose, e.g. sweets, cakes, biscuits, chocolate and soft drinks. Not only are these foods low in magnesium but may increase the amount that is lost in the urine.
- Avoid drinking too much alcohol – more than one or two units per day – as this too will lead to a loss of magnesium in the urine.

- Don't drink more than two or three cups of coffee per day. A lot of coffee might reduce the amount of magnesium absorbed, or increase the amount lost in the urine.
- Eat plenty of foods rich in protein especially meat, fish poultry and eggs. Vegetarian proteins may not be quite as good as others at helping the body retain magnesium.
- Some mineral waters contain appreciable amounts of magnesium and this can be another way of improving your daily intake of this mineral.
- Finally do not make use of strong laxatives which, by causing diarrhoea, can lead to a loss of both magnesium and potassium. Magnesium supplements themselves can be used as a laxative if you are suffering with constipation.

MAGNESIUM SUPPLEMENTS – TABLETS OR INJECTIONS

Though the trial of magnesium in patients with chronic fatigue gave magnesium by injection this should not be necessary as a routine. There are a number of different magnesium tablets available. A suitable dosage for correction of deficiency is between 200 and 600 milligrams per day for an adult and it is common for patients to be prescribed magnesium oxide or carbonate forms. These may not always be well absorbed, and magnesium aspartate, gluconate or amino acid chelate can be tried instead. Magnesium tablets are best taken divided up into two or three doses through the day and can be taken with meals or on an empty stomach.

Treatment should be for at least six weeks and may need

to be for six months if tablets are used and response is slow. Depending on circumstances it may be prudent to continue with a small daily dose of magnesium by mouth in the longer term.

Two other nutrients have also been shown to raise a reduced red cell magnesium level. They are high doses of vitamin B6 – 200 milligrams per day – and the trace element selenium at a dosage of 200 micrograms a day. Selenium acts as an anti-oxidant, protecting tissues from wear and tear and perhaps helps to improve the distribution of magnesium to the cells. The effect of vitamin B6 is explained in Chapter 11 on Fatigue and Premenstrual Syndrome.

CAN I JUST TAKE SOME MAGNESIUM?

Magnesium used to be one of the most popular self-administered supplements along with iron and calcium. It was used, and still is, as a laxative in the form of Epsom salts, which are magnesium sulphate, and in a variety of indigestion preparations because of its mild acid neutralising properties. They were rightly popular during the last century and the first half of this one because they were effective and extremely safe, though newer drugs and preparations have largely replaced them.

Magnesium salts can be dangerous if the kidneys are diseased because any excess of this mineral cannot then be excreted. This is rarely a problem but could occur if someone took large amounts and had undiagnosed kidney disease. Under more usual circumstances, if too much magnesium is taken by mouth then the most likely effect is diarrhoea. Diarrhoea might also develop gradually in someone with true magnesium lack who, after taking oral supplements for several weeks or months, notices a loosening of their motions. This is because the body no longer needs the amount that is being consumed and as a consequence less is absorbed from the gut with the unabsorbed magnesium passing through and stimulating the bowel.

So magnesium is really quite safe to take but if taken without some kind of blood assessment then some people with fatigue may be taking it unnecessarily and others might not take an adequate amount.

Fatigue and the B group vitamins

Despite the fact that there is significant evidence to show that there is a relationship between a deficiency of B vitamins, fatigue and mental symptoms, little attention has been paid to them. This omission is beyond my comprehension.

The B group or B complex vitamins are a related group of seven main water-soluble vitamins. Their characteristics and their effects on the body are closely inter-related and if there is a lack of many of them it can produce fatigue.

Let us first look at the general properties of this fascinating group of essential nutrients before we consider each one in more detail. The main properties of the group are as follows: they are all water soluble and, with the exception of vitamin B12, they are not stored to any great degree in the body. Most of them are essential to the series of steps in the body's metabolism that leads to the release of energy from carbohydrates and fats from the diet or from body stores.

They have a crucial role in the formation of red blood cells, the healthy functioning of the brain, nervous and muscular systems and the working of the immune system which helps us fight infection.

Though severe deficiencies are relatively rare there is substantial evidence that mild or moderate deficiencies do occur in well-defined situations that are relevant to people with chronic fatigue states. The factors that lead to deficiency also often result in several of the vitamins of this group being deficient rather than just one.

So much for the group, what about individual performances? Undoubtedly deficiencies of both vitamin B1 (thiamin) and vitamin B12 are the most capable of producing severe fatigue, but their lack is usually accompanied by a characteristic collection of other sometimes dramatic health problems. Some doctors and nutritionists argue that as these severe deficiency states are both rare and have such specific characteristics they have little relevance to chronic fatigue states. However, as we will see, mild fatigue and other minor physical and mental symptoms can be amongst the early symptoms of mild or moderate B group deficiency problems which might never fully progress to more severe and more easily recognised ill-health. Thus they may pass unrecognised.

FOOD SOURCES OF B VITAMINS

The B vitamins can be found in a wide variety of foods: cereal products, e.g. bread and fortified breakfast cereals, meat, milk, cheese, fish, nuts and seeds. Dairy products are also a particularly good source of vitamin B2 (riboflavin). Oranges and some green vegetables contain good amounts of folic acid, but vitamin B12 is not found in any vegetable-based foods – only in meat, eggs and dairy products.

FEATURES OF DEFICIENCY

Vitamin B1 (thiamin)

Insomnia, irritability, anorexia, weakness and fatigue. Thiamin is essential for the release of energy from carbohydrates and its lack results in a build up of lactic acid (a chemical by-product of that energy release) which produces painful and easily fatigued muscles.

More severe deficiencies cause heart muscle weakness, tender calf muscles, loss of sensation in the arms and legs, double vision, loss of recent memory, mental disturbance and even brain damage.

At risk groups   Alcoholics, the elderly, anyone with repeated vomiting, anyone with a poor diet with a high intake of sugar-rich foods or alcohol, those with depression, anxiety or other mental symptoms. Deficiency can develop rapidly, within days or weeks in ill individuals.

Vitamin B2 (riboflavin)

Sore tongue, cracking at the corners of the mouth, redness and greasiness at the sides of the nose and possibly a burning feeling in the feet. There are no really serious symptoms.

At risk groups   The elderly, alcoholics and malnourished individuals. Other more serious deficiencies are likely to be present too.

Vitamin B3 (niacin or nicotinamide)

Dry, scaly, red or darkened skin on the face, neck, backs of the hands or other areas of the body exposed to light.

Diarrhoea, depression and other mental symptoms can develop.

At risk groups Alcoholics, the elderly, people eating a very poor diet or with serious digestive problems.

Vitamin B5 (pantothenic acid)

Fatigue, weakness, muscle cramps and tingling in hands or feet. No serious ill-health results and significant deficiency is exceptionally rare.

At risk groups Alcoholics or people eating a very poor diet.

Vitamin B6 (pyridoxine)

Apathy, poor appetite, depression, irritability, sore tongue, cracking at the corners of the mouth, redness or greasiness of the skin at the sides of the nose and occasionally numbness or tingling in the hands or feet.
  Mild deficiency is of uncertain significance and seems to occur in a proportion of the normal adult population.

At risk groups People with anxiety, depression or other mental symptoms, alcoholics, the elderly, and some people taking the oral contraceptive pill or hormone replacement therapy that contains oestrogen.

Biotin

Anorexia, depression, muscle pain and fatigue have all been reported to occur together with a greasy red skin rash.

At risk groups Deficiency is extremely rare. It can occur in those who consume large amounts of raw eggs as they contain an agent that blocks the absorption of biotin. Alcoholics and those with other severe B vitamin deficiencies are also at risk.

Folic acid

Anorexia, insomnia, forgetfulness and irritability. Sore or burning tongue, recurrent mouth ulcers, weakness or numbness in the arms or legs and possibly generalised weakness and fatigue.

Anaemia eventually develops, resulting in a pale appearance, shortness of breath and fatigue.

At risk groups The elderly and excessive alcohol consumers (yet again) and those with anxiety, depression or other mental symptoms. Patients with severe digestive problems or taking long-term anti-cancer, anti-epileptic or antibiotic medication.

Mild deficiency is of uncertain significance and is apparently common in the UK adult population especially women of child-bearing age and those who are unemployed or from poor circumstances.

Vitamin B12

Very gradual onset of weight loss, weakness and *fatigue*. Sore tongue, recurrent mouth ulcers, poor resistance to infection and a wide variety of mental changes including depression and memory loss can occur. Anaemia can develop resulting in a pale appearance, shortness of breath and worsening fatigue.

At risk groups   Strict vegans (those who do not consume any animal products). People who have had part or all of the stomach or end portion of the small bowel removed after surgery and people with other digestive disorders. Those aged fifty or more who can lose the ability to absorb vitamin B12 from the diet without realising it. This is more common in people with diabetes, thyroid disease or rheumatoid arthritis and in the close relatives of those with these conditions or with proven vitamin B12 deficiency itself.

Deficiency of this important vitamin develops very slowly over several years after a stomach operation or only after following a strict vegan diet for many years.

SUMMARY

To put this rather technical information into perspective, let me summarise the most important points:

- Certain B group vitamins when deficient can produce fatigue. This is particularly true for vitamin B1 (thiamin) and vitamin B12.
- Fatigue and other minor symptoms may occur due to B group deficiencies without a full picture of severe deficiency being present.
- Though the risk groups for severe deficiencies of these vitamins are well known, milder deficiencies may easily pass unnoticed.

Case History

Harry Boar

Harry had several problems, only one of which was fatigue. He had been a very fit man for all of his life, but now at the age of seventy-eight he had noticed a number of problems. For two years or more he had been troubled by a sore tongue, with loss of taste. Original investigations had shown that he was not anaemic, and no oral or dental problems could be found. His fatigue had crept on gradually over the last two years, and in the last six months he had noticed that he had lost half a stone in weight and that he was becoming increasingly unsteady on his feet.

One look at this tongue told me that there was something wrong. The surface of the tongue was smooth with a loss of the healthy cells in the taste-buds from its surface. His balance clearly was poor and he had difficulty standing still with his feet close together and his eyes shut. These features were very suggestive of vitamin B12 deficiency, and his blood level was 60 nanograms per litre which was well below the normal range of 280–750. A number of other nutrients were also low, but this probably occurred as a secondary effect of the lack of appetite and weight loss that had been caused by the vitamin B12 deficiency. This had come on slowly, and classically produces a progressive and severe anaemia called pernicious anaemia. But interestingly, in Harry's case, he was not actually anaemic. Doubtless this would have developed if it had not been treated.

A bowel specialist helped with further investigations, and treatment with vitamin B12 produced a marked improvement in his tongue symptoms, weight loss and fatigue.

Vitamin B12 deficiency is a rare cause of fatigue, but should be considered, particularly if you are older and particularly if you have experienced an unexplained weight loss, loss of balance or mental deterioration.

HOW COMMON ARE B VITAMIN DEFICIENCIES?

Ideally it would be useful now to tell you about the results of a detailed survey of several hundred sufferers of chronic fatigue whose nutritional state had been carefully assessed. Alas no such study has been published nor, to the best of my knowledge, has ever been attempted. However, there have been many assessments of different groups in the population and they can be divided into several categories: the normal population; those with mental complaints; the elderly; alcoholics; and other groups. The lessons learnt from these studies can be usefully applied to some people who suffer with chronic fatigue.

Vitamin B deficiency in the normal population

There have been several relevant studies but none that have looked at all of the B group of vitamins. The most detailed study in the United Kingdom is the *Dietary and Nutritional Survey of British Adults* (age sixteen to sixty-four years). In this survey, the results of which were published in 1990, dietary assessments of the intakes of all of the major vitamins were made but only vitamins B2-riboflavin, vitamin B12 and folic acid were assessed by blood analysis.

The main results relating to vitamin B showed that many adult men and women in the UK had excellent intakes of all of the B group vitamins. However, the intakes for some of these vitamins were low or borderline in a significant percentage of women, most notably the younger age groups and the unemployed.

The results of the blood analyses of folic acid, like those already discussed on iron, revealed that a substantial percentage of the healthy normal population were mildly deficient. In all, 13 per cent of men and 23 per cent of women had values that could be considered to be deficient.

There have been some other surveys in healthy groups both in the UK and elsewhere that give us a more complete picture. A survey of healthy adults in Northern Ireland also found that a high percentage of men and women had folic acid levels in the blood below the lower end of the accepted normal range. Also the results for vitamin B12 were at a level associated with damage to the nervous system in between 1 and 2 per cent of the adult population in this same group.

Vitamin B6 assessments have been made in two groups of women attending a private well-women centre in London. Even in these well-off women, 15 per cent were found to have low levels of vitamin B6 which indicated mild to moderate deficiency, but that there was no difference between those with premenstrual problems and those without.

Folic acid intakes and blood levels have been assessed in the US population as part of the previously mentioned National Health and Nutrition Examination Survey with findings very similar to the UK. Blood analyses on 10 per cent of the 11,166 nineteen to seventy-four-year olds in the original survey were performed and showed that one in twelve had a low red cell folic acid concentration which the authors concluded '... remains a problem in poor and institutionalized elderly individuals, in low-income women, and in adolescents.' This echoes the findings in the UK.

Unfortunately in these and other studies with similar findings there has been no real attempt to determine what actual effect these laboratory-diagnosed deficiencies have on physical or mental health. This is likely to depend on the quality of the rest of the diet, how long the deficiency has been present and the overall level of health. From a large amount of human and experimental work such deficiencies could easily influence physical energy levels, mood and resistance to infection.

Vitamin B deficiency in the elderly population

This doesn't give any cause for comfort either. In brief the independent 'free-living' elderly often eat very well and have a good nutritional intake. However, being dependent upon others, being institutionalised, being seriously unwell or just being poor means that deficiency is much more likely.

Studies in the UK and Republic of Ireland have discovered deficiencies in most of the B vitamins in a not insignificant proportion of elderly patients. The actual effect of these deficiencies was not obvious except in the extreme cases. Other studies conducted in the healthy elderly in the US have shown that those with the lowest blood levels of vitamins B2, B12 and vitamin C performed less well on tests of non-verbal abstract thinking. Additionally a similar pattern was obtained for vitamins B2 and C in relation to tests of memory. These effects were only noticeable in those whose blood results were in the worst 5 to 10 per cent of the population. These sorts of blood results would be expected more frequently in less prosperous or more unhealthy communities.

There is also evidence that correction of these deficiencies by giving vitamin B complex can improve mental state. In summary, being deficient in one or more of some of the B vitamins can effect your powers of thought. It can also affect your mood as we will see next.

Vitamin B deficiency in psychiatric populations

There is no question that severe deficiencies of vitamins B1, B3, B6, B12 and folic acid can have a profound effect on mental state producing anxiety conditions, depression, dementia or schizophrenia, though this is rare. The more relevant questions are how common are mild to moderate deficiencies of these vitamins in those with psychiatric complaints, and does giving vitamin B supplements to them improve their mood?

Studies of vitamin B deficiencies in the psychiatric population have concentrated on vitamins B1, B6, B12 and folic acid and the findings essentially mirror those in the elderly. At the forefront of this research in the United Kingdom has been Dr Carney at Northwick Park Hospital, London. His studies have shown that in-patients with a diagnosis of anxiety, depression or schizophrenia had a 50 per cent chance of being deficient in one or more of vitamin B1 (thiamin), vitamin B2 (riboflavin) or vitamin B6 (pyridoxine). Depression was particularly associated with vitamin B2 or B6 deficiencies. Additionally about one-third of psychiatric in-patients are lacking in folic acid and a small percentage in vitamin B12.

Together with some colleagues from his own hospital and from King's College Hospital in South London, Dr Carney has conducted a very careful trial of a specialised form of folic acid in those with depression or other mental problems. Giving folic acid when compared with placebo resulted in a small improvement after two months which increased after four and then six months. Those who had received folic acid had had a greater degree of improvement both in their mental symptoms and rate of return to a normal social life. Only a few of these patients had a deficiency of folic acid severe enough to produce anaemia or other blood changes.

The implication is that the common finding of mild folic acid deficiency without anaemia, which seems to occur in some 30 per cent of people with mental illness and 10 to 20 per cent of the normal population, may be having an adverse effect on their mental state and sense of well-being. This may be quite relevant to chronic fatigue states in view of the overlap between this and depressive symptoms.

Vitamin B deficiency in other populations including post-viral syndrome

It is worth a look at the prevalence of vitamin B deficiencies in other groups.

A detailed assessment of vitamin B levels in a group of hospital-based patients has been made by Dr Carroll Leevy and others in New Jersey, USA. A random survey was made of 120 patients with medical, surgical or psychiatric problems, aged twenty-five to ninety years and from relatively poor backgrounds. All had a detailed laboratory assessment of their vitamin levels and 45 per cent were found to be low in folic acid, 31 per cent in low in vitamin B1, 29 per cent low in vitamin B3 (nicotinic acid), 27 per cent low in vitamin B6 (pyridoxine), 15 per cent in vitamin B5 (pantothenic acid), 12 per cent deficient in vitamin B2 (riboflavin), 10 per cent low in vitamin B12, and 1 per cent low in biotin. Mild deficiencies of other vitamins, including vitamins A, E and C were also found – a pattern rather similar to that in the elderly. The relationship between these deficiencies and symptoms was not assessed. But again there is no cause for complacency about those who are seriously ill.

The same group of researchers also looked at the incidence of vitamin B deficiencies in alcoholics, with similar findings. The risk of vitamin B deficiency rose substantially with an increasing level of damage to the liver.

Unfortunately, there are no equally detailed studies of vitamin B complex levels in those with chronic fatigue or post-infective syndrome. Indeed the only relevant publication I know of where the vitamin B status of patients has been assessed again showed a high prevalence of mild folic acid deficiency. Professor Jacobson and colleagues at the Department of Haematological Medicine at the University Clinical School, Cambridge, measured the level of folic acid in the serum in 260 patients with a recent viral or other chest infection with another organism called mycoplasma. An astonishing 60 per cent were found to have values below the lower end of normal! Deficiency was less likely in those who had had influenza and more likely in those with Epstein-Barr (glandular fever) virus or an acute unspecified viral infection that had produced a rash. In view of the influence of folic acid on many aspects of immune function as well as the nervous system these findings give substantial cause for concern. Perhaps we should reconsider the policy of some doctors of yesteryear. They used to give their elderly and debilitated patients who had recently had a bad infection a course of vitamin B or multivitamins. I think that we should add the poor and those with a below average diet to that list.

It is worth noting that in December 1992, the Department of Health in the United Kingdom recommended all women planning a pregnancy 'should take a daily dietary supplement of 0.4 milligrams [400 micrograms] of folic acid.' This was to help reduce the risk of birth abnormalities such as spina bifida in the offspring of mothers depleted in this vitamin. So much for the UK diet.

Trials of vitamin B supplements in fatigue

Despite all the foregoing evidence, there are extraordinarily no comprehensive trials of vitamin B supplementation in those complaining with fatigue or related physical or mental problems!

You may well ask why, and that in itself deserves another chapter. Firstly, the medical profession's awareness of mild and severe vitamin deficiency is poor. The common belief that most physically or mentally ill patients are not nutritionally deficient simply indicates the educational deficiencies in the believer.

Secondly, most vitamin supplements are relatively cheap and because they cannot produce the kind of profit that many pharmaceutical products can, research in this area does not receive the funding from industry that it deserves from the medical and scientific point of view. Unfortunately, until trials have been conducted into the effect of vitamin B supplementation in appropriate groups (including people with fatigue), we cannot truly assess how significant a laboratory-diagnosed nutritional deficiency is in establishing it as a (treatable) cause of fatigue.

Two small relevant studies have been conducted, one in a group of patients with fatigue who were given vitamin B12 injections, and the other in the group of elderly depressed patients who were given vitamin B complex.

Vitamin B12 supplementation in fatigue

In 1973, Drs Ellis and Nasser from Kingston Hospital, London, published the results of a small trial of vitamin B12 supplementation in a group of fatigued patients who had no clinical evidence of any vitamin B12 deficiency. Vitamin B12 was the last major B vitamin to be discovered and isolated in the 1930s. Since that time it had earned a reputation as a 'tonic'. It was most usually given by injection and its red colour probably enhanced the doctors' and patients' belief that it was doing some good. It has long been known that the majority of vitamin B12 given by doctors in the UK was not for the correction of an actual deficiency but as a tonic. This was a popular treatment during the 1960s and 1970s, but became ridiculed in the late 1970s and 1980s. The only proper study to assess its effects has been that of Ellis and Nasser.

They took a group of forty-five patients and staff at the hospital. Their major complaint was tiredness. They all had a normal physical examination, were not anaemic, nor deficient in vitamin B12 or folic acid. They were all offered treatment with a placebo or with vitamin B12 by injection at a dosage of 5 milligrams twice weekly for two consecutive weeks. Then after a two-week gap they were given the other treatment, either vitamin B12 or the placebo without knowing which.

The response was determined by self-assessment. Twenty-eight people completed the study. Those who had received placebo in the first two weeks showed a favourable response when they then received vitamin B12 in the second period. The other group who received vitamin B12 in the first period initially showed some improvement and in the second treatment phase with placebo showed no deterioration or improvement. Vitamin B12 at the dosage given would last for many months in the body. The improvement in symptoms was greatest in the categories 'general well-being', 'appetite' and 'happiness'. Fatigue and sleep problems did not improve so greatly.

The results of this study are almost unbelievable. Could the 'irrational' giving of vitamin B12 injections to all those fatigued and exhausted patients who required a tonic back in the 1940s, 1950s, 1960s and 1970s have been correct? We won't know until a repeat of this pilot study, as it was termed, is conducted. In the meantime, there certainly is no harm to giving vitamin B12, which is a cheap treatment, for a trial period of a couple of weeks at this may be all that is required to determine who might respond to this simple approach. It is possible that the increased amounts of vitamin B12 do genuinely have a stimulating effect upon the nervous system or other aspects of metabolism.

More recently, Dr Iris R. Bell and colleagues in the Department of Psychiatry and Geriatrics in Boston, USA, have looked at the effect of giving vitamin B1, B2 and B6 at a dosage of 10 milligrams each, to fourteen geriatric in-patients with depression. Some received a placebo and some these B vitamins, both in addition to standard antidepressant medication. Those receiving the vitamins showed some modest improvements in ratings for depression and tests of learning ability compared with those who received placebo. The authors concluded, 'These findings offer preliminary support for further investigation of B complex vitamin augmentation in the treatment of geriatric depression. It would also be interesting to conduct similar trials in younger patients with depression and in those with fatigue.' In other words, the doctors felt more research in this area would be well worth the effort.

Taking vitamin B supplements

Ideally, all those suffering with chronic fatigue syndrome should have some assessment of the adequacy of their diet. The risk of vitamin B deficiency increases substantially in people with a poor appetite or experiencing weight loss, in those who consume more than four units of alcohol a day, have a history of digestive disorders, or if depression is a significant feature of their fatigue. Unfortunately, tests to measure B vitamins other than vitamin B12 and folic acid are not widely available and they tend to be relatively costly. Provided vitamin B12 and folic acid deficiency have been excluded, which is relatively easy, using the appropriate and available blood tests, it is perfectly reasonable to try a course of vitamin B complex containing approximately 10 milligrams of vitamins B1, B2 and B6, and 50 milligrams of vitamin B3. You can buy these easily over the counter or they can be prescribed by your doctor.

In view of the slow response to vitamin B supplementation in the trials already conducted, supplements should probably be taken for up to six months before any final decision is made about the response to treatment. If there is no benefit, little has been lost. If there is some improvement, you should take care to ensure that your diet can continue to supply these and other nutrients, and either the supplements should be stopped or continued at a more modest level. This is a matter for judgement by both you and the doctor.

There are few hazards or dangers from taking vitamin B complex supplements at this sort of dosage. But if you are on drugs for Parkinson's disease you should check with your doctor before taking products containing vitamin B6. There is also a risk that if someone is unknowingly deficient in vitamin B12 and takes B vitamins containing folic acid, they may actually increase the risk of damage to the nervous system. This is a rare situation but I have seen this nearly happen on one occasion. Again, careful assessment by your doctor and measurement of vitamin B12 and folic acid levels will prevent this from occurring. Certainly, if you have tried taking vitamin B complex and symptoms of fatigue or muscle weakness do not improve or worsen, then you should check with your doctor without delay.

Fatigue and other nutrients

We have considered iron, magnesium and the B vitamins in detail because of the theoretical and practical evidence of their role in causing fatigue and other physical and mental symptoms. There are, however, many other vitamins, minerals and essential nutrients that are necessary to the health of the body and in particular have an influence on the function of muscles, the functioning of the immune system or have an effect on mood.

In this chapter the remaining vitamins and most of the essential minerals will be looked at in brief, giving some indication of their importance to health, the likelihood of deficiency and their relevance to chronic fatigue.

THE VITAMINS

Vitamin A

This exists in two forms; retinol derived from animal products and beta carotene which, as its name suggests, is

found in carrots and other red, yellow and green vegetables.

Vitamin A has particular effects upon the eyes and also
the skin. Deficiency of vitamin A in the Third World is still
a serious and easily preventable cause of blindness, but it
rarely occurs in Western countries. Mild deficiency of
vitamin A can occur in people losing weight because of
digestive problems, in the ill, elderly and alcoholics.

The first symptom is poor night vision – which can also
be caused by zinc deficiency. The functioning of the
immune system is affected by vitamin A and deficiency in
elderly patients has been shown to increase the ease with
which infecting bacteria stick to the lining of the lung.
Vitamin A also influences the body's ability to fight
infections once they are established. I have found borderline blood levels of vitamin A in a few patients with chronic
fatigue, but it is uncertain how significant this is to their
fatigue.

Supplements of vitamin A or multivitamins containing
vitamin A should not be taken by women who are pregnant
or are intending to become pregnant unless they are under
medical supervision. This is because recent reports suggest
that excess vitamin A in pregnancy may have an unhealthy
effect on the developing baby.

Vitamin D

Vitamin D is a vitamin with hormone-like properties. Most
of the vitamin D in our bodies is actually formed by the
action of sunlight on the skin which turns a derivative of
cholesterol into a chemical which is then metabolised
further in the liver and then the kidney, resulting finally in
active vitamin D.

The main actions of vitamin D are to encourage the

absorption of calcium from the gut and the movement of calcium into and out of bone. It also has a modest effect on the function of the immune system (and lack of vitamin D in children produces rickets which is not relevant to this book). In older patients deficiency can occur in those deprived of sunlight, such as old people who are institutionalised or who rarely go out of doors.

Like vitamin A, too much vitamin D can be harmful and dosage should not exceed the Recommended Nutrient Intake of 2.5 micrograms per day.

Vitamin E

This fat-soluble vitamin has been associated with many popular myths. One of its main actions is to limit the toxic effects of oxygen upon healthy tissues. Oxygen can interact with healthy tissues to produce powerful chemicals called free radicals which may cause tissue damage, and these may be relevant to inflammation and the development of cancer. Vitamin E, together with vitamin A and other nutrients, may help limit the production and effect of free radicals.

Vitamin E is found widely amongst vegetable foods, especially green leafy vegetables, nuts and vegetable oils. Deficiency is extremely rare but not unknown and can occur in those who have serious digestive problems resulting in weight loss, and in certain rare blood disorders. Deficiency can affect the blood, and the nervous and immune systems. Reduced blood levels have been recorded in ill elderly people and supplements of vitamin E in the elderly may, at times, act as an immune stimulant.

Normal requirements are in the region of 6–10 milligrams per day, and doses of up to some fifty times this amount have been shown to have a modest effect on certain functions of the immune system. Whether this produces any real benefit to the patient or not is uncertain.

Vitamin K

Vitamin K is another fat-soluble vitamin which is mainly found in green leafy vegetables. Some is synthesised by the healthy bacteria in our own digestive systems. Deficiency is extremely rare and can result in a delay in the blood clotting after an injury. But lack of this vitamin has no obvious effects upon mood or the immune system of relevance.

Vitamin C

Vitamin C, also known as ascorbic acid, is found in fresh fruit and vegetables but is easily destroyed by cooking or if food is kept hot for a long time before it is eaten.

Intakes in Western societies are on average very good. In the UK the average intake is between 60 to 70 milligrams per day for adults, with only a small percentage of the population consuming 20 milligrams or less. As little as 5 milligrams of ascorbic acid a day is enough to prevent the actual development of scurvy.

Early mild deficiency, however, can occur more easily and causes depression, hypocondriasis and hysteria before the features of scurvy develop. Men seem to need more vitamin C, probably because of their large muscle bulk, as do smokers who break down vitamin C more quickly in the body. The elderly and those who live in institutions are most at risk of developing modest vitamin C deficiency because of the over-cooking of vegetables and lack of fresh fruit in the diet.

Many convenience foods are low in vitamin C. For example, some commercially produced apple pies contain, according to the manufacturer's analysis, no detectable amount of vitamin C. The process of manufacture, storage and cooking have destroyed the vitamin C contained in the apples and in the extra vitamin C added whilst it is being made.

A person's vitamin C requirements can also be increased in acute illness, infection, cancer or where there is an increased need for tissue repair or healing, such as in burns or after an operation.

Vitamin C has many roles. It is required for optimum strength of blood vessels, the metabolism of cholesterol, the detoxification of drugs and other compounds by the body and it has some influence on the immune system. It is also involved in the production of carnitine which, though it is not a vitamin, is a chemical required for the transport of energy-producing fats into muscle cells. Muscles have a high demand for fat as a source of energy. When vitamin C levels are low or borderline, reduced muscle function can follow.

This might explain the classic description by Dr James Lind, the British naval physician who gave us one of the first descriptions of scurvy and its treatment in 1753. He observed that the sailors suffered from, 'listlessness to action, or an aversion to any sort of exercise' in the early stages of scurvy.

Two studies on experimental scurvy conducted in the United States have demonstrated that fatigue is indeed an early feature of experimental vitamin C deficiency which can also cause dull aching muscular pains in the legs.

Studies on vitamin C and fatigue

Despite the enormous popularity of vitamin C as a supplement very few studies have been conducted on vitamin C and fatigue. There are only two studies of relevance.

Drs Buzina and Suboticanec from the Institute of Public Health, Zagreb in the former Yugoslavia looked at the effects of supplementing vitamin C together with vitamin B2 and B6 in a group of adolescent boys aged between thirteen and fifteen, many of whom had evidence of mild mixed vitamin B and C deficiencies. Those who received supplements over a three-month period when compared with a control group who did not receive any supplements showed an improvement in the maximum uptake of oxygen during exercise – a good measure of work capacity. A part of this improvement may have been due to a modest improvement of haemoglobin and iron levels in those receiving the vitamins because vitamin C encourages better absorption of iron from the diet. The improvement also related to the increase in blood levels of vitamin C when a mild deficiency was being corrected but not once the blood levels were in the normal range. So correcting a deficiency is important but taking extra may not help muscle function further.

In conclusion, a supplement of vitamin C might be useful for people who are at risk of deficiency and are suffering fatigue. This would include those:

- With a history of poor diet, especially smokers, the elderly and people living in institutions.
- With active chronic infections – viral or bacterial.
- On long-term drug therapy with steroids, tetracycline antibiotics and aspirin. These drugs increase the need for vitamin C.

If you are experiencing fatigue without evidence of an active or continuing infection and are well fed, then you are unlikely to have even a marginal vitamin C deficiency.

If you do decide to take a supplement of vitamin C the dosage should probably be in the range of 200–500 milligrams per day, which is some three or four times the average daily intake in most Western populations. This amount is necessary to build up depleted stores of the vitamin. If you are going to experience benefit it should be evident within six to eight weeks. If you do have a deficiency of vitamin C it is likely that you may also have modest deficiencies of B vitamins, iron and possibly other minerals. You should take this into consideration when choosing food and supplements.

Coenzyme Q10

Coenzyme Q10 is not a vitamin but a chemical involved in energy production. It can be derived from the diet or made in the body from two amino acids in conjunction with vitamins B and C. Dietary sources include most nutritious animal and vegetarian foods. High levels in the human body are mainly stored in the kidneys, liver and heart. Levels fall with increasing age, if the diet is poor, with liver disease and in certain rare genetic disorders.

Low levels might occasionally be of relevance to fatigue because Coenzyme Q10 has the ability to help move chemicals that take part in the energy-producing activities in all cells of the body. It may also have chemical uses in certain rare metabolic problems, and in those who experience muscle fatigue as a result of certain cholesterol-lowering drugs. It has also been studied in a group of healthy adults who, after taking 60 milligrams of Coenzyme Q10 daily for four to eight weeks, were observed to improve their work capacity by between 3 to 12 per cent. How relevant this is to the more general population of people with fatigue, either following a episode of infection or chronic inactivity is uncertain. Again this is another good reason for ensuring a good diet, adequate intakes of protein from either animal or vegetable sources and also adequate amounts of vitamins B and vitamin C. Coenzyme Q10 can be found in health food shops – but it is very expensive.

MINERALS

Calcium

This mineral is found mainly in bones, but is widely distributed throughout all the cells in the body, including muscles. The main source of calcium in the diet is from dairy products, approximately 50 per cent in many Western countries with the remainder coming from vegetables, nuts, seeds and bread. White bread is fortified with calcium in the United Kingdom.

Absorption of calcium is limited by phytic acid which is a chemical found in bran and to a lesser extent in wholemeal bread. If the dietary intake of calcium is poor, particularly if this is combined with a lack of physical exercise it can result, after many years, in osteoporosis – a thinning and weakening of the bones. This may only be evident later in life especially in women after the menopause when the lowered production of oestrogen from the ovaries accelerates the rate at which calcium is naturally lost from the skeleton.

This deficiency of calcium does not have any known effect on mood or the immune system. Disturbances in the way calcium is used in the body certainly can occur, not as a result of dietary inadequacy, but as a result of hormonal disturbances. A high or low blood calcium – hypo- or hypercalcaemia – are important potential causes of fatigue and muscular problems. Chapter 5 on fatigue caused by Physical Illness on pages 53–86 goes into this in more detail.

Potassium

Potassium is another mineral which with sodium is one of the most important minerals controlling the salt and water balance in the body. Phosphate, magnesium, sodium and potassium all play an essential role in the actual structure of the body including that of bones, muscles and individual cells, and help to maintain their shape as well as their function.

Potassium is widely distributed in foods especially fruit and vegetables, and a dietary lack is rare unless the diet is low in these foods. If potassium levels are too high or too low it can have an adverse effect on muscle function, leading to early muscle fatigue and weakness. Interestingly, low levels of potassium inside the cell greatly reduce the ability of many cells to produce protein and grow properly. Conversely a high level of potassium also interferes with the function of muscles. Levels of potassium in the blood rise naturally during intensive physical exercise and this appears to be one of the factors that limits very intense physical activity after a few minutes, which is the body's way of preventing exhaustion.

Blood levels of potassium can be low in alcoholics, in people taking older style diuretics (water tablets), in the elderly and as a result of some drugs including some anti-asthma drugs. Low levels of potassium rarely occur outside these situations. Fatigue may be the only evident symptom that a person is lacking in this mineral.

High levels of potassium may be found in older patients with mild or severe kidney failure especially if they are using a salt substitute excessively, or taking potassium saving diuretics or the anti-arthritis drug indomethacin.

Potassium is, therefore, a classic example of a nutrient where too much or too little has an adverse effect on muscle function. This is not surprising as an adequate balance of both sodium and potassium are necessary for the generation of minute electrical currents in the muscles which are essential to muscle contraction and relaxation, that is the muscle's ability to work. A check on your blood potassium and magnesium levels is advisable if you are suffering with chronic fatigue. A disturbance of potassium or magnesium can also be due to a variety of hormonal conditions.

Sodium

Sodium is the sister mineral to potassium, and deficiency is rare in Western diets as it is frequently added to preserve or flavour foods. Fresh fruit and vegetables are low in sodium.

High intakes over a lifetime are associated with increased risk of high blood pressure whilst low levels of sodium may produce muscle weakness, easy fatiguing and cramps. Low sodium levels are often associated with hormonal disturbances, kidney disease and use of diuretics (water tablets) in older people.

Low levels can be detected by a blood test. The treatment usually involves limiting your fluid intake rather than adding extra sodium salt to your diet. Supplements of magnesium may improve sodium and potassium balance and this demonstrates how these important minerals interact.

Zinc

Zinc, like iron, is a trace element which has many specific and important functions. The necessity of zinc to human health was only recognised in the early 1960s when deficiency was found to cause growth retardation and delayed sexual development in adolescent males, plus a whole host of problems in a group of newborn infants who weren't able to absorb zinc properly. Disturbances in the immune system and poor resistance to infection were soon recognised as features of severe zinc deficiency.

Good food sources of zinc include meat – especially red meat – offal, vegetarian proteins, wholemeal bread, and to a lesser extent, modest amounts are found in most other wholesome foods. Zinc is now thought to play a part in some sixty enzyme and chemical reactions throughout the body, as well as having an influence on maintaining the health of genetic material – the DNA – in the cells. Again, severe deficiency is relatively rare and usually only happens where a person has an extremely poor diet, in alcoholics, or in people with very poor absorption of nutrients due to digestive problems. Milder forms of zinc deficiency may occur sporadically in healthy people, for example in some children, in elderly people who are ill, and may be particularly likely to occur at times of physical stress. Pregnancy, breastfeeding, burns, infections and recovery from an operation may all cause some degree of zinc deficiency unless stores or intake are very high.

The effects of modest deficiency may include:

- Slight reduction in resistance to infection.
- Poor wound-healing.
- Reduction in taste sensitivity.
- Poor night vision – like vitamin A deficiency – and the development of a red, greasy, scaly rash on the face.
- Slight disturbance in brain and hormone chemistry.
- A lowered sperm count in men.

It is certainly possible that people who have a low zinc intake might be more likely to suffer with recurrent minor infections. Sucking zinc lozenges has been shown to help shorten the duration of infective sore throats. This may be because the zinc has a local anti-viral effect in the throat, or perhaps because of a mild immune-stimulating effect.

High-dose zinc supplementation in the elderly has also been shown to act as an immune stimulant, but again the clinical significance of this is uncertain. It is certainly worth correcting even a mild zinc deficiency especially if you have recurrent infections that are a contributory cause of your fatigue.

In 1992, a trial using multivitamins, zinc and other minerals in well-fed elderly people was conducted by Professor R.K. Chandra from Newfoundland, Canada. He gave a group of elderly patients vitamins and minerals at a dosage close to the normal daily intake. Many of them had laboratory evidence of mild nutritional deficiencies which were corrected by the supplement. During the year-long study, those who received the supplement had half the number of days troubled by acute infections and half the usage of antibiotics compared with those who did not.

Thus taking zinc and other nutrients may hasten recovery from infections in individuals with nutritional deficiencies. However, the value of zinc supplements alone in people with chronic fatigue is uncertain. It certainly would be appropriate to assess the level of zinc in some patients with chronic fatigue especially where a severe or repeated infection(s) play a part.

A word of caution: large amounts of zinc may have an immune-suppressing effect, which is probably undesirable. Dosages of zinc should not normally exceed more than 30 milligrams, about three times the normal daily intake.

Copper

Copper is an essential element which is widely distributed in most wholesome foods. Deficiency is extremely rare and occurs only in people who have a disturbance in copper metabolism. It does not cause fatigue. Taking copper supplements is inadvisable.

Selenium

Selenium is in some ways the nutritional partner of vitamin E. It too counteracts the toxic effects of oxygen by limiting the damage caused by free radicals to healthy tissues. It is widely distributed in most wholesome foods. Severe deficiency is rare but it is known to occur in certain parts of China where it results in heart disease. A mild deficiency may have subtle influences on the body's ability to respond to infections and other health problems. Its value as a supplement in the majority of situations including fatigue is uncertain.

Chromium

Chromium is an extraordinary trace element. It has a very specific function which is to enhance the action of insulin – a hormone which is vital to the processing of sugar by the body. Blood and tissue levels of chromium decline with age and its lack may be associated with rising blood cholesterol levels and an increased risk of developing diabetes in later life. It has no obvious influence on the immune system or mood. A few people who have low levels and eat a poor diet may have poor blood sugar control which might be a cause of fatigue, see page 188 (hypoglycaemia). Again, it too is widely distributed in wholesome foods.

Iodine

Iodine is yet another trace element with a very specific function. It is essential for the production of thyroid hormones. Deficiency is rare but has occurred in the past in areas far away from the sea like Switzerland, the Mid-West in the United States and Derbyshire in England (hence the term Derbyshire neck to describe goitre). Increasing the variety of vegetables and seafood in your diet, as well as eating salt fortified with iodine will improve your iodine levels. There are no obvious known effects on fatigue except in cases of extreme deficiency when thyroid function is reduced and there is marked swelling of the thyroid gland in the neck. It is inadvisable to take large amounts of iodine or kelp without medical advice.

Other trace elements

Manganese, vanadium and cobalt and perhaps a few other trace elements may have some minor function in human biochemistry. Deficiency states have not been described in medical research. They are easily provided by eating a wholesome diet.

Fatigue and premenstrual syndrome

Why a chapter on fatigue in premenstrual syndrome? Well, fatigue is a common premenstrual symptom and there is considerable overlap between some of the successful treatments for PMS and chronic fatigue syndrome.

The first description of fatigue as part of premenstrual syndrome was in 1937 with the publication by Drs McCance, Luff and Widdowson from King's College Hospital, London, of their article 'Physical and Emotional Periodicity in Women'. McCance and Widdowson were, in fact, two of the foremost nutritionists of their day and at that time they also took a considerable interest in menstrual problems.

The authors conducted a detailed study of 167 women who kept daily symptom diaries for an average of five menstrual cycles. Interestingly they found that fatigue was the commonest symptom occurring before and during menstruation, being reported twice as often as depression, breast pain and tearfulness. The cause for fatigue just before or around menstruation has never been clearly determined, but other work has thrown considerable light on to premenstrual syndrome in general.

PREMENSTRUAL SYNDROME – WHAT IS IT?

Premenstrual syndrome is a collection of various symptoms, either physical or mental, that characteristically occur for a few days, or up to two weeks before a period and improve with, or shortly after, the onset of menstruation. Common symptoms include mood swings, irritability, depression, headaches, breast tenderness, weight gain, abdominal bloating and clumsiness, loss of sexual interest and fatigue. Many researchers during the 1960s and 1970s attributed premenstrual syndrome to a hormone imbalance, but no studies have consistently shown any significant hormonal imbalance in women with PMS.

NUTRITION AND PREMENSTRUAL SYNDROME

There now seems to be a considerable connection between PMS and nutritional factors. Researchers at Westminster Hospital in London have shown that the level of iron in the blood – but not haemoglobin – falls sharply four days before the onset of menstruation, and stays low during the period. It is clearly connected with the loss of blood. Despite this work being known for over twenty years, no study has been carried out to determine whether these physiological changes in iron level are associated with physical or mental symptoms, especially those of PMS.

Most of the more recent interest has centred on vitamin B6 (pyridoxine) which has been a popular treatment for PMS. But, like hormonal imbalance, women with PMS are

not more prone to vitamin B6 deficiency than those
without, and only minor disturbances in the way vitamin
B6 is processed by the body have been detected in PMS
sufferers. Though vitamin B6 (pyridoxine) has been studied
in many past trials in PMS, the results are conflicting. This
was certainly the conclusion of a Dutch review of thirteen
vitamin B6 trials in premenstrual syndrome.

Dr Guy Abraham, a leading researcher from the United
States, has with colleagues looked at the levels of magnesium
in women with premenstrual syndrome. You may recall that
magnesium is important in the body's chemical reactions
involved in energy production, muscle function, nerve
function and is also involved in the action of some hormones. In Dr Abraham's study it has been shown that
reduced levels of magnesium in the red blood cells have been
found in women with PMS when compared with healthy,
non-sufferers. Too often such reports are one-off. However,
we ourselves at the Women's Nutritional Advisory Service
together with colleagues in Sussex and in London have
confirmed this finding in two separate studies, which again
showed that red cell magnesium levels in PMS sufferers are
some 20 to 25 per cent lower than the healthy norm.

An Italian group headed by Dr Facchinetti from the
University of Modena, studied the effect of administering a
large dose of magnesium to women with premenstrual
syndrome. Only in this way can scientists really determine
the importance of this mineral in premenstrual syndrome. In
their study, treatment with placebo tablets produced no
change in magnesium levels, nor any improvement in
premenstrual symptoms, whereas those who received
magnesium experienced a significant rise in the level of
magnesium, and a substantial reduction in their level of
premenstrual symptoms. The beneficial effect of magnesium
was particularly noticeable on symptoms of depression and

low energy levels. Unfortunately, fatigue itself was not assessed independently.

Other studies combining magnesium with vitamin B6 and multivitamins have again shown a modest reduction of premenstrual symptoms in three out of four double-blind, placebo-controlled trials (i.e. trials where neither the patient nor administering doctor know whether the drug they are receiving is the active one being tested or a harmless placebo). It seems that a mild magnesium deficit is part of premenstrual syndrome, therefore, just as it can be part of chronic fatigue syndrome, and that some sufferers with both complaints would respond to supplementation.

Evening primrose oil has been used as a treatment for premenstrual syndrome. Its benefit is mainly confined to improving premenstrual breast tenderness. It is probably best combined with a low-fat, high-fibre, high-protein diet which has also been shown to be of benefit in premenstrual breast tenderness, and such a diet is likely to improve the intake of many nutrients, including magnesium.

CHRONIC FATIGUE SYNDROME AND PREMENSTRUAL SYNDROME

If you are suffering from chronic fatigue and notice that it is worse before a period, then some or all of the above may well apply to you. Ideally, your level of magnesium in red blood cells should be measured. This is a relatively simple test which can be undertaken by most medium-sized hospital laboratories. A lowered level would strongly suggest that a trial treatment with magnesium, perhaps combined with multivitamins, would be a good idea.

Very often it is better also to combine this type of

treatment with dietary change. The Women's Nutritional Advisory Service suggests you make improvements to your diet which follow on from those first expounded by Dr Guy Abraham. The general dietary recommendations for PMS sufferers are:

- Reduce your intake of sugar (sucrose) and 'junk' foods. This includes sugar added to tea and coffee, sweets, cakes, chocolates, biscuits, puddings, jams, marmalade, soft drinks, ice cream and honey.
- Reduce your intake of salt. This includes salt added to cooking and at the table. Most salt, however, comes from salty foods which should be avoided, e.g. salted nuts, cheese, kippers, many tinned meats and fish products, and preserved meats and other meat products, e.g. bacon, ham, sausages and pâtés. Excess salt may cause fluid retention which might displace magnesium and indirectly worsen your fatigue.
- Reduce intake of tea and coffee. Consume no more than one or two cups of tea, and one cup of coffee per day. Caffeine aggravates anxiety and may bring on migraine headaches. Use herbal teas instead, and one to two cups of decaffeinated coffee per day.
- Eat a good portion of green vegetables or salad daily. These are high in many vitamins and minerals useful in the treatment of premenstrual syndrome.
- Limit your intake of animal fats. This is particularly true if you are over-weight. Avoid fatty cuts of meat, trimming all visible fat from meats. Meat products such as sausages and pâté are usually rich in animal fat and are best avoided. Allow up to half a pint of milk, normal or skimmed, per day and 4 oz of cheese per week – more if you are vegetarian.
- Use good quality vegetable oils and margarines. Sun-

flower or safflower seed oils should be used for cooking or for making salad dressings. A good quality sunflower seed soft margarine should be used, rather than butter or hard margarines.

- Limit your use of tobacco and consumption of alcohol. Cigarettes and alcohol have many harmful effects upon general health, and decrease the levels of many vitamins and minerals in your body. Ideally you should not smoke at all, but if you are a heavy smoker reducing this to five per day or less would be acceptable. Alcohol should be no more than one unit per day (one unit = one glass of wine = one pub measure of spirits = half a pint of normal strength beer). Less alcohol should be consumed if you are over-weight or have severe premenstrual problems.

- Eat plenty of nutritious, wholesome foods. Good foods include lean meat, poultry without the skin, eggs, fish, all green vegetables, salads, wholemeal bread, nuts and seeds. All the above foods are rich in either protein or vitamins and minerals. Many are also rich in fibre, particularly vegetables, salads, nuts, seeds and wholemeal bread. Fruit is also rich in fibre, but it is not as nutritious as vegetables. Avoid eating bran unless it is essential for treating constipation. Bran blocks the absorption of many nutrients and is not as good a source of fibre as vegetables and fruit.

- Eat regularly. Eat three good meals a day. Make sure that you start the morning with a good breakfast containing protein, e.g. a good quality fortified breakfast cereal or an egg. Lunch and supper should likewise contain protein from either meat, fish, egg, nuts, seeds, beans or other vegetarian sources. It may be helpful to have snacks at mid-morning and mid-afternoon, particularly if your energy level fluctuates. Good snacks include fresh fruit, a sandwich or a small portion of nuts and dried fruit.

- Lose weight if you are obese. An unhealthy diet or being over-weight may affect not only your general health but also your hormonal balance, and thus contribute to premenstrual syndrome. Though losing weight may take a long time, it can be of long-term benefit. Also, eating a healthier diet may reduce a future risk of both heart disease and cancer.
- Be patient. It may be better for you to make the changes in your diet gradually, but do persist with them. The improvement in your premenstrual syndrome may well take up to three months before you experience the full benefit.

Finally, premenstrual syndrome can also be eased by regular aerobic, i.e. sustained fitness rather than strength improving, physical exercise. This is clearly a tall order for someone with fatigue, but gradually building up your level of physical activity can not only help your energy levels but also your premenstrual symptoms. This we will come to later. The full nutritional programme of the Women's Nutritional Advisory Service is outlined in the book *Beat PMT Through Diet* by Maryon Stewart (published by Vermilion).

OTHER TREATMENTS FOR PREMENSTRUAL SYNDROME

As well as using diet and nutritional supplements there are a number of other treatments which can be helpful. Certain types of painkillers are useful for both period pains and PMS. The oral contraceptive pill does help lessen some women's premenstrual symptoms though for others it can make them worse. Hormonal preparations are of limited value. There is no good evidence that pessaries of progesterone are effective and the very powerful hormonal treatments, though effective, cannot usually be used in the long term.

If you have severe premenstrual problems and bad period pains or irregular or heavy periods then you should consult your family doctor, as occasionally gynaecological problems may be responsible which will not necessarily respond to nutritional treatments.

Fatigue and allergy

The idea that allergy to food or to other agents can produce fatigue is not new, but it is a concept that is not widely appreciated. First of all, let us define a few terms. Allergy comes from two Greek words, which simply mean altered reaction. Its usage is best confined to reactions either to a food, chemical, cosmetic or inhalant (such as a pollen) that involves changes in the blood or white blood cells in an identifiable way. Many other types of adverse reactions occur without changes in the immune system involving blood proteins or white blood cells. These events are best termed intolerances.

Common examples of genuine allergies include hay fever, asthma and eczema. Here, reactions to grass pollen or other plant pollens in the case of hay fever and asthma, or to cosmetics in the case of eczema, result in localised inflammation and irritation to the nose, lung or skin. These reactions usually only happen with a specific substance termed an allergen, and come on after a delay of minutes or occasionally days, and last for several hours or days before resolving. If the allergen – allergy-causing compound – is present all the time, then symptoms can persist for weeks or months. If the allergen is present only at certain times of the year, then this is termed a seasonal allergy as in the case of hay fever in the summer or reaction to mould spores in the late summer and autumn.

CONDITIONS CAUSED BY ALLERGIES AND INTOLERANCES

During the 1980s considerable controversy surrounded this subject. Reports from leading organisations in the United States and from the Royal College of Physicians in the United Kingdom, as well as many popular books and medical and scientific articles, have addressed this subject. Overall, there seems little doubt that a wide variety of conditions can be caused by allergy either to food, inhaled allergens or contact with various chemicals.

For our purposes it is important only really to consider those conditions caused by food allergy or intolerance. These are best divided into two groups. It should be carefully noted that all the conditions in both categories can also be caused by a variety of factors other than allergy.

Conditions definitely caused by food allergy or intolerance

This includes eczema, asthma, allergic rhinitis (hay fever lasting the whole year round), coeliac disease, irritable bowel syndrome, unexplained diarrhoea, some cases of ulcerative colitis and Crohn's disease (which sometimes can be a cause of chronic fatigue), migraine headaches, urticaria (nettle rash), hyperactive behaviour in children and rheumatoid arthritis.

Case History

Eric Poulson

Eric was a twenty-year-old textile design student who had always been very fit, but during his college course had noticed that his concentration and energy levels began to wane.

There had been no great illness that would have accounted for this. He had been checked over by his general practitioner following a trip to Africa, and routine investigations into possible tropical diseases were all satisfactory. Even so, he still felt fatigued. Another problem was that he had had mild eczema on his face and neck which required the use of steroid creams from time to time.

He drank ten pints of beer a week and for as long as he could remember he had Marmite on toast for his breakfast every morning. I thought that his eczema might be caused by a food sensitivity to something that he was consuming regularly, such as bread, dairy products, beer or the Marmite. Within two days of stopping these foods the eczema improved markedly, and reintroducing only the Marmite and beer produced a return in his eczema. Avoiding these and making some other minor changes to his diet kept his eczema at bay and he felt that his energy level and powers of concentration improved. He also had a low zinc level in the blood which might have had an influence on his skin condition and resistance to infection.

Minor degrees of ill health may be viewed as a problem to those who have particularly physically or intellectually demanding jobs. Eczema can indeed be caused by food allergies and occasionally this can be to yeast.

Conditions occasionally caused by food allergy and intolerance

This is a much wider group and includes conjunctivitis, depression, non-migraine headaches, epileptic fits, recurrent mouth ulceration, vaginal discharge, chronic cough, fluid retention, nephrotic syndrome (a type of kidney disease), palpitations, infantile colitis, mild gastro-intestinal blood loss in infants, failure of infants to grow normally, constipation, glue ears, muscular aches and pains, idiopathic thrombocytopenic purpura (a blood condition) and fatigue.

Case History

Teresa Smith

Teresa was a dynamic woman with a high-powered job in the City of London. Her powers of concentration and stamina had been reduced over the last two years following repeated minor chest and dental infections. She had also been troubled by several episodes of vaginal thrush that required appropriate treatment with antibiotics from her GP. She was left with mild fatigue, an occasional feverish feeling, a tendency to diarrhoea and increasing anxiety over her state of health. A blood test had shown a mildly abnormal liver function and evidence of a recent probably viral infection.

Nutritional investigations were normal apart from moderate vitamin B1 (thiamine) deficiency. I strongly suspected that her bowel symptoms had been precipitated by her infections. Avoiding a variety of foods, notably milk, cream and other dairy products, cutting down on sugar and avoiding yeast-rich foods made a big difference. Taking supplements of vitamin B as well as making the changes in her diet increased her energy level, and she seemed to experience fewer coughs and colds.

It is quite possible that Teresa was unable to digest milk sugar (lactose). This can occur after bowel infections and is more likely to occur in people of Eastern European, Indian or Asian origin. Teresa's mother was, in fact, from Greece.

I advised Teresa that if she was not able to tolerate milk and dairy products later on, that she should probably take a calcium supplement providing 500 milligrams per day, and to make sure that she ate plenty of other calcium-rich foods such as sardines, nuts, seeds, green vegetables, beans, peas and lentils. This advice is particularly important for growing children who may have to avoid dairy products for some reason or another, and for women of menopausal age (to reduce the risk of osteoporosis – bone-thinning disease). Lactose and other food intolerances may, however, settle with time, and sometimes supplements of vitamin B may help improve the situation.

So where does fatigue come in in the scheme of things?

ALLERGIC TENSION-FATIGUE SYNDROME

The concept that allergic reactions could produce feelings of tension and fatigue was first put forward by some of the early American allergists in the 1930s and 1940s. An initial theory proposed that repeated challenging by a food, or possibly an inhalant, to which one is allergic 'exhausts' the body's immune system. This is rather simplistic and probably incorrect. Many doctors have noticed that people with the allergic conditions mentioned above who also have fatigue may experience considerable improvement not only in their underlying condition but also in the reduced energy level when the food or other allergen causing their problems is avoided. Indeed, a number of popular organisations have suggested that people with chronic fatigue syndrome should consider excluding a variety of foods from their diet to help determine whether allergy or intolerance is contributing to their symptoms. This seems a reasonable suggestion, especially if an obvious allergic condition is also present. Whether those with fatigue without any other features of allergy or intolerance would benefit from the exclusion of foods is uncertain.

Scientific evidence

This rather controversial viewpoint is supported by some very interesting and recent evidence from Iceland. Dr Arnason and colleagues investigated 200 normal healthy individuals who had been selected from the electoral register and were therefore considered to be representative of the normal adult population. A number of blood tests were performed for anaemia and for evidence of allergy to a wheat protein using a very sensitive test for anti-gliadin antibodies by a method termed ELISA (enzyme-linked immunosorbent assay). My apologies for the science, but this is an important detail as other tests may not be so sensitive or so accurate. The surveyed group were also asked about a variety of symptoms including fatigue.

A high percentage tested positive for anti-gliadin antibodies. Of the original two hundred, thirty-two (or 16 per cent) were positive and the results of their other blood tests and symptoms were compared with a group of those whose test was negative. The 16 per cent who appeared to have some reaction against wheat protein had slightly lower levels of haemoglobin and iron though they weren't actually anaemic. The researchers thought that the sensitivity to wheat was great enough in some of this group to have resulted in damage to the lining of the gut causing a reduction in the amount of iron that was absorbed from the diet.

An unexpected finding was that those with a degree of wheat protein sensitivity experienced more 'headaches', 'unexplained bouts of diarrhoea' and 'fatigue' than those in whom the test had been negative.

This was the first good evidence that fatigue in the normal population may be linked to allergy. This work doesn't actually prove that an allergy to a food was the cause of the fatigue – we would only know this by altering the diet of those with fatigue and seeing what the effect was. My own experience is that in some people with chronic fatigue, especially those with other symptoms of food allergy or intolerance, a trial of a diet excluding foods that commonly cause adverse reactions is well worth trying.

Case History

Josephine Lynton

Josephine Lynton was a twenty-eight-old social worker who was suffering with chronic fatigue and abdominal swelling following an episode of mumps. She admitted that she had been under a considerable amount of stress at work and was also in the process of being ostracised by her family because of her intention to marry outside her faith.

She had previously had what she described as unlimited energy and used to swim most days. By the time I saw her she had been ill for some nine months and had seen many doctors in an attempt to find the cause of the symptoms that were 'ruining her life'. She was unable to work as she could not be up for more than half an hour without experiencing severe discomfort, abdominal bloating and fatigue. She had begun to follow an exclusion diet at the suggestion of her general practitioner and noticed a considerable improvement. It appeared that she was allergic to wheat, oats, barley and rye and this was in fact confirmed by the specialised blood test. She continued to exclude these grains from her diet, took a multivitamin and mineral supplement and extra supplements of magnesium which helped her constipation.

After six months her abdominal bloating had disappeared and her energy levels gradually improved. She did get married and has since had several children. She remains well and attributes the secret of her success to following her diet, taking regular exercise, avoiding stressful situations and making plenty of time to relax. However, her inability to tolerate wheat and other grains persists.

WHAT IS AN EXCLUSION DIET AND HOW DOES IT WORK?

An exclusion diet is simply a diet that excludes one or more foods for a specified period of time. There are many different types, ranging from those that exclude only one food or a food group such as milk and other dairy products, to the very harsh diets where everything but a few foods such as lamb, pears, rice, carrots and water is avoided.

The use of these diets is really best considered in three phases.

- An exclusion phase.
- A re-introduction phase.
- A long-term therapeutic phase.

The exclusion phase is followed for between one and three weeks and the symptoms are carefully monitored by the patient and therapist. At the end of this first phase if there is an improvement then it is reasonable to suppose that this could have resulted from excluding a food that was causing or contributing to the symptoms. This won't be known until the next phase. If there is no or only very minimal improvement then that is the end of the trial. Occasionally it is wise to try a second different exclusion diet but there must be good grounds for so doing.

During the re introduction phase each food or group of foods is brought back into the diet at intervals of between three to seven days. Symptoms continue to be monitored carefully so that if there is any deterioration then the relationship to specific foods can be determined. A reaction to a food can occur within minutes but more often it is after several hours or even days. If this occurs the food or foods that have most recently been brought back into the diet are then excluded again, hopefully with a return to the previous level of improvement. This part of the diet can be very tedious and time-consuming but taking care at this stage will save considerable time and trouble in the end. By proceeding carefully, a list of suspect foods can be compiled which if necessary can be re-introduced again at a later stage to check if the adverse reaction was real or apparent.

The third phase is, strictly speaking, the treatment phase when foods known or just suspected of causing or aggravating symptoms are avoided for several months at a time. At the end of this or sometimes during this phase it may be appropriate to try the foods being excluded once again and watch for any reactions. This whole process can take several months and expert guidance is often necessary along the way.

There are, however, certain hazards and limitations of exclusion diets and it is necessary to consider these.

The 'down' side

Firstly, it should be said that these diets should only be undertaken in someone with chronic fatigue if they have first been thoroughly assessed for any other identifiable cause of fatigue. Beginning on such a diet when there is some other underlying illness is potentially dangerous and will almost certainly not result in any improvement but instead may encourage the patient to lose contact with the doctor.

Secondly, an exclusion diet is *not* a treatment for any condition including fatigue. These diets are initially used as a means of determining whether or not any foods cause or aggravate the complaint in question. Once these foods are identified they are then avoided on a short- or long-term basis while making sure the rest of the diet is well balanced. Exclusion diets should not be followed for months or years as they are not usually a nutritionally well-balanced or adequate diet.

If after reading through this book you feel it would be worth trying to isolate foods or other dietary factors that may be aggravating your symptoms, you can follow the instructions on pages 254–71. For those with severe fatigue who are contemplating trying an exclusion diet it would be essential to discuss this with your own doctor first.

Fatigue and Candida

Candida is the name of a yeast species which commonly infects the skin or mucous membranes. An infection is termed candidiasis or more properly, candidosis. There are several types of Candida organisms, the most common being Candida albicans.

The reasons that this common yeast merits a chapter in a book on fatigue are several. Firstly, it has been proposed that infection with Candida in various forms has been a cause for chronic fatigue. This was first put forward by Drs Truss and O'Shea from the United States. Secondly, this view has been strongly challenged by medical authorities in the US. Thirdly, much of the popular information about Candida, in my opinion, is misleading, and if my experience is anything to go by there seems to be a genuine need for the record to be put straight.

HOW COMMON IS CANDIDA?

Candida is a highly successful yeast organism. It rarely causes serious illness, except in those who are extremely ill with a very damaged immune system. More usually, it causes minor infections. A high percentage of the normal population, between 20 per cent and 40 per cent, have Candida residing in their mouths or other parts of the gastro-intestinal tract without it causing any significant ill health. Candida may also be present in the vagina of 11 per cent of non-pregnant women, and in 25 to 30 per cent of pregnant women. Invasion of tissues produces local and occasionally more widespread symptoms.

FACTORS THAT MAKE CANDIDA INFECTION MORE LIKELY

Actual infection of the tissues rather than just surface colonisation with Candida can come about because of:

- Damage to local tissues.
- Usage of antibiotics – this allows an increase in the numbers of Candida organisms in the gut as healthy bacteria, which usually keep the Candida in check, are reduced by antibiotics.
- A weakened immune system, e.g. in patients with cancer, leukaemia or HIV infection, especially if receiving drug treatment. A few people have a very poor natural resistance to Candida infection.
- Diabetes. The increased levels of sugar in the blood and other tissues encourage the growth of Candida.
- Warmth and moisture. This encourages the growth of all yeasts, and skin infections are more likely to occur in women and men who are overweight or who wear tight underclothing made of synthetic non-absorbent material.
- Nutritional deficiencies. Deficiency of iron with or without anaemia, is a known predisposing cause.

Other nutritional deficiencies may also be relevant.

- Steroid drugs, and possibly powerful tranquillisers like chlorpromazine which may also cause a greater risk of Candida infection.
- Hormonal problems. Under-active thyroid or adrenal glands or a low blood calcium can all lower resistance to infection with Candida.
- Periods of physical challenge, for example during infancy, old age and pregnancy.
- The oral contraceptive pill. This is occasionally a risk factor. The newer lower dose oral contraceptives seem to be much less of a problem than their high-dose predecessors.
- Having an intra-uterine contraceptive device (coil).

It is also possible, but not certain, that dietary factors may contribute to colonisation of the mouth and gut with Candida albicans. Perhaps a high intake of sugar and refined carbohydrates in the diet may be inadvisable in this respect, but at present this is not quite clear.

INFECTIONS CAUSED BY CANDIDA

Most of the infections are superficial. The organism Candida, instead of just living on the surface of the skin or mouth, invades the tissues, but usually only the first few layers. This produces inflammation, soreness and irritation, which then results in the majority of symptoms.

What to look out for

Mouth   Red sore gums and inflamed lining of the mouth or tongue, with white deposits, are typical of Candida infection. It can also cause cracking at the corners of the mouth, a red patch in the middle of the tongue and occasionally more severe problems. A white or furred tongue that is not sore or inflamed is not due to significant Candida infection.

Vagina   Vaginal thrush is a common problem. Typically soreness and irritation of the vagina and vulva and a white sticky discharge are the classic features of Candida. The picture, however, may vary as there are often bacterial infections at the same time. Many women are silent carriers of Candida albicans.

Skin   Nappy rash in infancy is, to a large degree, caused by Candida. The rash has a typical appearance: a red blotchy rash with smaller red spots at its edge suggests a yeast organism invading the outerlying tissues. The rash is normally localised to the groin and the area between the buttocks. Women may notice a rash under the breasts and occasionally in the armpits, and this may also be the first obvious sign of diabetes, especially in older patients.

Nails   An infection of the nails occasionally occurs in nurses and housewives who often have their hands in water. Typically, there is a dull red painful swelling at the side of the nails which persists for weeks rather than days.

The bowel   The presence of Candida in the bowel is a much harder situation to evaluate. First of all, some 20 to 30 per cent of the normal population will have Candida in their bowel from time to time, usually without any ill effect. Problems may flare up after a course of antibiotics. Researchers at the Albert Einstein College of Medicine in New York, led by Dr Paolo Danna, have found that diarrhoea following the use of antibiotics is often associated with a substantial increase of Candida in the bowel. There has been evidence to suggest that Candida overgrowth also occurs in some patients with irritable bowel syndrome and possibly Crohn's disease, and there have been reports of these conditions responding to treatment with anti-fungal agents, either alone or in combination with other medication. There is the real possibility that large amounts of Candida in the gastro-intestinal tract might pass into the bloodstream, or produce changes in blood chemistry in a way that might produce a variety of symptoms distant from the gut. Drs Truss and O'Shea in the United States suggested that this was perhaps the cause of a whole host of symptoms, including fatigue, headache, mood swings, irritability, digestive symptoms, abdominal bloating, wind, diarrhoea, poor concentration and memory.

Other researchers have indeed found an association between Candida albicans and urticaria (nettle rash) and possibly between eczema and psoriasis in occasional patients. It is asking a lot to believe that a whole host of general symptoms could be caused by infection by one particular organism. But the popularity of the concept was enhanced by the publication of two best-selling books in the 1980s, *The Missing Diagnosis* by Dr C.O. Truss in Birmingham, Alabama, and *The Yeast Connection: A Medical Breakthrough* by Dr W.G. Crook (Professional Books, Jackson, Tennessee, 1984). The popularity of these two books, supported by anecdotal reports, rather irritated the medical establishment in the US. Two trials published in 1989 and 1990 went some way into investigating the claims and concepts put forward by Truss and Crook.

Trials of anti-Candida therapy in treating fatigue

The first publication, by Drs Renfro, Feder, Lane, Manu and Matthews from the University School of Medicine in Connecticut, assessed 100 patients with chronic fatigue. Eight of those who 'thought' that their fatigue was due to chronic candidiasis were assessed further, and seven of them were considered to have a psychiatric diagnosis!

Of the remaining ninety-two patients with chronic fatigue, fifty-nine were also considered to have an underlying psychiatric diagnosis. None of the patients who thought they had a Candida infection were found to have a physical illness. Each had been carefully assessed by standard examinations and a battery of blood and other tests. In both groups, 90 per cent of patients had evidence of good normal immunity against Candida and none of those with a self-diagnosed Candida infection had clinical or laboratory evidence which showed an active Candida infection at the time of examination.

No firm conclusions can really be drawn from this publication. Certainly, there was no strong evidence that supported the theories put forward by Truss and Crook that chronic hidden yeast infection or colonisation of the bowel is a common cause of fatigue.

1990 saw the second relevant publication by Dr Dismukes and colleagues from the Birmingham School of Medicine at the University of Alabama in the United States. This was entitled 'A Randomised, Double-blind Trial of Nystatin Therapy for Candiasis Hypersensitivity Syndrome'. In brief, forty-two pre-menopausal women who met the conditions for chronic Candida syndrome and who had a history of Candida vaginitis were entered into the study. Each was given in different sequences, four different types of treatment with the anti-fungal agent Nystatin.

This included Nystatin by mouth and vaginally; Nystatin by mouth alone with a vaginal placebo (dummy tablet); Nystatin vaginally with oral placebo (dummy tablet); and double placebo for both oral and vaginal use. No dietary changes were made. Many symptoms were monitored including vaginal symptoms and a wide variety of physical symptoms, including fatigue. By approaching treatment in this way, the researchers could compare whether treatment with oral Nystatin, which would be expected to kill off yeast organisms in the gut, influenced symptoms of general well-being.

Vaginal symptoms did appear to improve whenever vaginal pessaries of Nystatin were used, as would have been expected, and irritation, burning and discharge improved significantly. There was some indication that abdominal symptoms also improved with oral treatment, as did irregularity of periods, but a whole host of general physical and mental symptoms did not improve significantly in the active treatments when compared with placebo.

An editorial in the same edition of the *New England Journal of Medicine* in which the study by Dr Dismukes and colleagues was published commented, 'The study by Dismukes and colleagues is a reasonable way to begin to sort out this issue. But it is only a beginning. Additional scientifically sound studies will be needed to determine whether this syndrome does or does not exist, and if it does, what the optimum treatment is for patients'.

This is fair comment. The study did not involve changes in diet or advice to avoid mouldy environments and the use of Candida allergy injections as had been advocated by Drs Truss and Crook. It may be that some of the more general physical symptoms would improve if these other therapeutic measures were included.

Case History

Sarah White

Sarah was a sixty-three-year-old housewife and part-time secretary. For many years she had taken sleeping tablets and tranquillisers and had bravely eased herself off these after ten years. Even though this was several years ago, she was still troubled by a wide variety of symptoms the cause of which was not entirely clear, though she had attributed this in part to being dependent on tranquillisers.

She experienced modest fatigue which didn't prevent her from doing her work but meant that each day was a struggle. There were generalised aches and pains that were worse on exercise and limited her walking and socialising. For the last few years she had also experienced bowel problems with a tendency either to constipation or diarrhoea, which at its worst was associated with mild abdominal discomfort. She had also been putting on weight, now to 79 kilos ($12\frac{1}{2}$ stones) and with this she had developed quite a bad thrush infection of the skin under her breasts. This responded only partially to a powerful anti-fungal agent prescribed by her GP. She clearly needed some further help.

Her GP had already performed a number of basic investigations to exclude diabetes and other conditions that might have brought about the thrush. However, her serum zinc was markedly reduced at 9 micromols (normal range 11.5–20). There was also evidence of vitamin B6 deficiency and a borderline red cell magnesium level. It is known that both vitamin B6 and zinc are essential in the body's fight against infection, and in particular, their deficiencies may bring about a thrush infection. Sarah took supplements of these and followed a weight-reducing diet which also excluded a number of foods that are known to trigger irritable bowel syndrome symptoms. Her weight fell from 79 to 73.5 kilos, her thrush cleared with a second course of anti-fungal treatment from her GP, and her bowel symptoms improved dramatically on avoiding a variety of foods. Because of her proven deficiencies, her GP was happy to prescribe the supplements for Sarah, which she continued with for several months before gradually tailing them off.

With these reductions in her physical symptoms and weight, her energy level improved. The cloud of ill health that she had once attributed to being on tranquillisers began to lift. It is interesting how a number of relatively minor problems combined together to produce general feelings of ill health, and that they responded so successfully to both conventional and nutritional treatments.

WHO WITH FATIGUE SHOULD BE TREATED FOR CANDIDA?

The treatment of Candida involves the use of an anti-fungal agent or agents, avoidance or correction of factors likely to bring on an infection, and sometimes dietary change. This approach may be worth considering if you have fatigue and also one or more of the following features:

- Proven Candida infection in the vagina or mouth – diagnosed by your doctor. This will require careful examination and usually swabs are taken and sent off to a laboratory for analysis.
- Urticaria (nettle rash or hives). There is excellent evidence from the late British dermatologist, Dr Robert Warin from Bristol, that sensitivity to Candida albicans is an important factor in about 26 per cent of patients with chronic urticaria, and that there may be a cross-

reaction between Candida and food yeast as well. Eradication of any infection with Candida albicans and the avoidance of yeast in your diet may be an important approach (see pages 259 and 267).

- Irritable bowel syndrome, characterised by abdominal bloating, discomfort, wind, diarrhoea or constipation or alternation between the latter two. Again, assessment must be made by a medical practitioner to exclude more serious bowel disorders. Over-colonisation with Candida albicans was suggested as a factor in IBS by Dr Holti, a skin specialist from Newcastle, as long ago as 1966. And yeast tablets, as a cause of abdominal upset and diarrhoea, was first reported in the *Journal of the American Medical Association* as long ago as 1944!

- Other ill-defined and allergic symptoms including eczema, asthma, urinary symptoms or digestive problems. However, this theory is based on anecdotal reports, some of which stretch back to those by a French physician, Jacques Sclafer from Paris in 1957.

So you can see there is nothing new about Candida albicans, nor the fact that it may produce not only local infections but a variety of more general symptoms. How much overlap there is with this in the chronic fatigue syndrome is unclear. It is noteworthy that the Candida albicans organism can itself actually suppress certain aspects of immune function. So the connection may be a significant one for some patients with proven Candida infections and chronic fatigue. In essence, the advice is if Candida is present, treat it; if it is not, look for some other cause.

Treating Candida

The mainstay of treating Candida involves:

- The correction of factors that are likely to bring on an infection.
- The use of anti-fungal agents.
- Advice about diet.

That said, a significant percentage of patients almost certainly improve spontaneously in view of the common nature of Candida infections and the fact that only very rarely do they cause serious disease.

Treating factors likely to bring on a Candida infection

Most of those already listed will be obvious when your condition is assessed and you have related details of your past medical history. Testing the urine for diabetes and the blood for iron deficiency are particularly relevant.

Anti-fungal treatments

There are now many to choose from. None is universally effective, but most produce an improvement in 80 to 90 per cent of cases. Agents include Nystatin, Amphotericin, Miconazole, Fluconazole, Itraconazole and Ketoconazole. Some are available as tablets, creams, shampoos, vaginal preparations and some for intravenous use for those with rare and severe life-threatening infections.

Oral treatment is often for a week, sometimes extending for as long as six weeks for those with recurrent Candida. Vaginal treatment can be given as a one-day, one-off dose which is sometimes very effective, but at other times prolonged treatment for two or three weeks may be necessary. Skin preparations often combine the anti-fungal agents with a small dose of steroid which helps reduce the inflammation and irritation. However, the usage of steroid ointments alone is ineffective and may lead to worsening and spreading of any fungal infection.

Dietary treatment

The majority of simple Candida infections do not require making any changes to your diet unless you are diabetic or eating a poor quality, nutritionally inadequate diet. If, however, you have bowel symptoms or urticaria (nettle rash) or other symptoms which suggest a true yeast intolerance you may well be helped by making dietary changes and avoiding yeast-rich foods (see page 259). Sometimes it may be prudent to limit your intake of refined carbohydrates, including sucrose – table sugar – glucose and all foods containing them. Additionally, some patients, particularly those with bowel symptoms and urticaria, may be allergic to or intolerant of a variety of foods or food additives, so an exclusion diet may be worth a try (see page 254).

Fatigue and associated minor conditions

There are a number of minor conditions that can occur by themselves or in association with chronic fatigue. Some of them respond well to treatment in their own right and therefore deserve special consideration as resolving them may help the associated fatigue.

It is perhaps worth reading through the list of minor conditions with a view to selecting the advice that may be appropriate for you. The conditions that I wish to consider are:

- Hypoglycaemia – low blood sugar.
- Day-time drowsiness.
- Hyperventilation – over-breathing.
- Headaches and migraine.
- Fluid retention.
- Fibromyalgia or fibrositis – muscle aches and pains.
- Restless legs syndrome.
- Snoring and sleep apnoea – temporary stopping of breathing.
- Irritable bowel syndrome.

- Low blood pressure.
- Obesity.

Insomnia or a disturbed sleep pattern are of particular importance and merit their own chapter (see page 206).

HYPOGLYCAEMIA

This term literally means 'low level of sugar in the blood'. The sugar in question is glucose, which is the sole source of energy for the nerves and brain. A lack can result in a sudden decrease in energy level, poor concentration, drowsiness and even coma. A slight excess produces no symptoms but sustained high levels are the hallmark of diabetes which is due either to a lack of the hormone insulin or to an insensitivity of the tissues to it. The glucose in the blood-stream is derived from the glucose and other sugars in our diet; from the breakdown of other complex carbohydrates found in vegetables, fruit and bread; and from the break-down of fats and protein from the diet and stored by the body.

Very low levels of glucose in the blood occur in certain rare medical conditions: liver disease, alcoholism and insu-lin-producing tumours, and often first show up when the patient in question has gone without food for a while.

Mild forms of low blood sugar may also occur as well in some relatively healthy people, some of whom have attributed their chronic fatigue to this condition. However, it is now thought that other aspects of body chemistry are also relevant.

The body responds to a low blood sugar by producing adrenaline, a hormone which raises the blood sugar but also increases pulse rate, blood pressure and causes sweating and feelings of anxiety and nervousness. These symptoms together with mild intermittent fatigue, drowsiness or poor concentration may occur with a very low blood sugar.

People who experience these symptoms if they miss a meal, or an hour or two after eating when the blood glucose level is falling after its initial rise, may require some investigation of their blood glucose levels. For the technically minded, a seriously low blood sugar is defined as 2.2 millimols per litre or less. It is most unusual for such levels to be recorded and if they are then the precise cause of it must be found. The normal range for blood sugar is from 3.5 to 6.5 millimols per litre, and thus there is a grey area of between 2.2 and 3.5. Some, but not all, researchers have found that those who experience a dip in blood sugar to these levels may experience mild mental or physical symptoms, but these findings are not consistent. It is more practical to consider that those of us who feel unwell if we miss a meal or after eating a meal are less robust than those who do not.

Physical factors such as obesity, our level of physical fitness, the balance of some essential nutrients (vitamin B, chromium and magnesium) and the type of diet we eat all influence blood sugar control. Furthermore, there are changes in circulation, blood pressure and in a host of minor hormones in the hour or two after a meal. Some of these changes are not well tolerated by the elderly, the infirm and those with health problems.

For most of those who experience swings in energy levels that seem related to food then the following practical advice should help the majority. If it does not then some further assessment may be necessary.

- Eat regularly – three meals a day with small snacks in between if necessary.
- Do not eat large amounts of sugar, sweet foods,

chocolate, cakes, soft drinks, honey, etc. They may cause a rapid rise, sometimes followed by a fall, in blood sugar and other changes to body metabolism.

- Eat plenty of complex carbohydrates, e.g. fruit, vegetables and also peas, beans, lentils and pasta. These cause relatively small rises in blood sugar. Wholemeal and white bread are rapidly digested and metabolised and in fact cause the same degree of rise and fall in blood sugar that a chocolate or candy bar produces.
- Having adequate protein intake in the diet will help improve blood sugar control. This means having meat, fish, chicken, eggs, dairy products or vegetable protein with each meal.
- Lose weight if you are over-weight. This helps blood sugar control.
- Do not drink large amounts of alcohol, especially on an empty stomach. This can certainly aggravate the situation.
- Avoid large amounts of coffee and tea, especially if you take sugar, as this may further destabilise blood sugar control.
- Take regular physical exercise. Being physically fit improves blood sugar control and this is perhaps the least of its benefits!
- Occasionally some nutritional supplements may help in the control of blood sugar, e.g. magnesium, chromium and possibly the B vitamins. These should normally be provided by a well-balanced diet.
- Take a rest after eating a large meal. This is particularly important for the elderly, those with heart problems and perhaps the very unfit.
- If particular foods seem to upset you regularly then avoid them. Genuine food allergy or intolerance can sometimes cause feelings of unwellness, fatigue and

other symptoms after a meal.

If physical symptoms repeatedly occur when you have not eaten for a while, despite the measures above, then check with your own doctor. People who have particularly poor blood sugar control may be at risk of developing diabetes or may have a metabolic problem requiring investigation. Equally if you continue to feel unwell after eating despite these measures then check with your doctor.

The principles on which the dietary recommendations above are based are included in the diets that appear in Part 2.

DAY-TIME DROWSINESS

Day-time drowsiness can also be a problem and complicate the picture of chronic fatigue. It can occur for a variety of reasons including an exaggerated response to eating a meal or true hypoglycaemia. Often it is physiological, that is occurring naturally in response to certain situations but there are other causes. Causes of excessive day-time drowsiness include:

- Lack of night-time sleep.
- Disturbed sleep because of night snoring (yours or someone else's!).
- Sedative drugs or a hangover from night sedation.
- Alcohol.
- After a meal, especially at lunch time.
- Boredom and lack of stimulation.
- Possibly as an adverse reaction to some foods.

For example, it is now known that there is a natural decline in alertness in the early afternoon following lunch. This effect is most noticeable in men and is influenced by the size and composition of the midday meal. Alcohol may certainly worsen this effect and tea and coffee, with their content of caffeine, may help minimise it. Perhaps some of those with chronic fatigue syndromes have an exaggerated response to this physiological variation of alertness during the course of the day. There seems no harm in having a catnap for thirty to sixty minutes if that is what is required at this time. This may be particularly useful for the elderly and those with chronic heart or lung disease. A siesta is not illegal in northern European countries and North America!

Another solution to those who experience a dip in energy levels after eating lunch or other meals is to go for a walk for ten or fifteen minutes. The change in surroundings, a breath of fresh air and mild exercise may provide a degree of refreshment that a catnap does not provide. Exercise has some beneficial and subtle effects on the function of the nervous system and its helpfulness should not be under-estimated.

Finally if you do experience severe day-time drowsiness, see your doctor. There is a rare condition called idiopathic recurring stupor – marked unrousable deep sleep for a few hours or days. This has recently been shown to be caused by the body producing its own home-made sedative which is chemically very similar to Valium and other benzodiazepine tranquillisers. It responds dramatically to a drug that reverses the effects of benzodiazepines.

HYPERVENTILATION SYNDROME

Hyperventilation means over-breathing. Its effects have been well known for many years, but in the last decade interest in it has increased considerably.

The function of the lungs is not only to take up oxygen,

but also to release carbon dioxide, a waste gas. Carbon dioxide is produced by the burning of carbohydrates, fats and proteins in the body to create energy, but it is not an entirely useless waste product. In fact the body requires a certain amount to maintain the correct acidity balance of the blood. Over-breathing results in a slight increase in the level of oxygen in the blood but a great decrease in the level of carbon dioxide. This can either happen acutely (suddenly) during a panic attack or almost imperceptibly on a chronic (long-term) basis. Classic symptoms of hyperventilation include tingling in the fingers and hands or feet, increased emotional sensitivity and exhaustion.

Good research work has clearly demonstrated that such a syndrome exists, but despite its similarity to chronic fatigue syndrome, researchers have not found hyperventilation to occur more commonly in patients with chronic fatigue. However, there certainly appears to be some overlap. A simple do-it-yourself test is to take twenty deep breaths and see if this provokes a return or aggravation of physical or mental symptoms. The fall in carbon dioxide concentration leads to a change in body chemistry with increased sensitivity to adrenalin and increased activity of the autonomic nervous system – the nervous system that controls blood pressure, circulation, bowel and bladder function.

Treatment involves explaining to a patient that there is a physical component to their mental and physical symptoms; breathing exercises to help re-establish control over breathing; and other measures to reduce anxiety, e.g. restricting caffeine, limiting stressful situations, gentle physical exercise and occasionally the use of anti-anxiety drugs or appropriate nutritional supplements. Some doctors have suggested that a lack of magnesium is important in hyperventilation syndrome. This has to be confirmed, although a recent report has suggested that it is effective in children with hyperventilation and neurological problems.

HEADACHES

Generalised headaches are an acknowledged feature of chronic fatigue states. Again they can have physical causes, or be associated with depression or stress. Generalised or tension headaches produce pain either over the whole of the head or localised in one area. They can vary from being dull to severe, occur daily or infrequently, be continuous or episodic (occur at intervals). If they are episodic, occur on one side of the head and are associated with nausea, vomiting and visual disturbance, then they are likely to be migraine.

There are also a variety of other types of headache, most of which do not have sinister causes. Lack of sleep, depression, neck and back problems, possible food intolerances, caffeine excess or caffeine withdrawal can all contribute to generalised headache, and may respond to measures that address these problems, such as simple painkillers and sometimes low doses of antidepressants which may have pain-relieving effects. Other causes of headaches include chronic sinus infection, dental problems, eye problems, high blood pressure and very occasionally neurological or hormonal problems. Anyone with chronic severe headaches should be examined carefully by their doctor, and this should include measurement of their blood pressure.

As well as changing and improving the diet, tension or migraine headaches can be helped by relaxation techniques, acupuncture, osteopathic manipulation and sometimes herbal remedies.

Migraine headaches

Migraine headaches are different from tension headaches in that they are episodic (they occur at intervals), often severe (though they can be mild) and are associated with visual disturbance, nausea or vomiting. It is now known that a variety of chemical and nervous system changes occur in the build up to and during a migraine headache. In the early part of the development of migraine, there are often warning symptoms such as flashing lights, tingling or other warning sensations. The headache classically develops on one side of the head and is often centred around the eye. With increasing intensity of the pain, nausea and vomiting often develop.

Increased sensitivity to light or noise are common accompaniments and drive the sufferer to retire to a darkened room to try and sleep it off. Very occasionally these symptoms can occur with little or no headache and then the diagnosis is confusing. The whole episode normally lasts a few hours or at its worst up to three days.

Normally there is a great sense of relief as the headache clears. Migraine headaches are episodic as a rule with a headache-free period of several days, even months, before the next attack. Curiously, migraine headaches do not appear to be more common in patients with chronic fatigue syndrome. Certainly, however, those who already suffer from migraine may notice an aggravation of their headache if they have developed fatigue.

Migraine headaches can be precipitated by lack of sleep; hormonal changes, especially in the week before a period; drugs, including the oral contraceptive pill; and dietary factors. Missing a meal may also be relevant. Dietary advice for migraine sufferers (known as migraineurs) is given in Part 2 of the book. Many sufferers already know that cheese, chocolate and wine may precipitate a headache.

These foods are rich in amines – a type of naturally occurring chemical – and many other foods also contain them. Colouring agents and wheat have also found to be common food triggers. Not all migraine headaches are triggered by food, but at least 50 per cent seem to be influenced by this.

If an attack is developing, simple painkillers taken early can be effective, as may breathing in and out of a paper bag to increase the level of carbon dioxide in the blood. Sometimes just going to bed and having an early night is all that needs to be done.

There are now a wide variety of drugs that may help reduce the chance of migraine headaches developing, if they are taken on a regular basis. They include low-dose anti-depressants and beta-blockers, as well as a variety of drugs that interfere with some of the chemical changes that occur in migraine headaches. For dietary advice for the prevention of migraine headaches see pages 241–3.

FLUID RETENTION – IDIOPATHIC OEDEMA

You may wonder what fluid retention is doing in a book on chronic fatigue. However, the two conditions co-exist and indeed overlap. Dr Anthony Pelosi and co-researchers from the Institute of Psychiatry in London, described a group of twenty-five women who were troubled by excessive fluid retention causing swelling of the feet, hands or abdomen. This condition is medically known as idiopathic oedema – literally swelling of unknown cause. When these women were compared with other gynaecological patients, they were more likely to complain of a variety of physical symptoms – fatigue, irritability, poor concentration, depression and anxiety – a pattern that should sound familiar to you by now. What is occurring here is that we are seeing patterns of symptoms in particular types of patients. The pattern may overlap greatly with premenstrual syndrome when there is a cyclical nature to these symptoms – getting worse before the period and improving with, or after, its arrival.

Typically, idiopathic oedema – fluid retention – was treated with intermittent or prolonged use of diuretics (water tablets). This is now considered inadvisable. Dr Graham MacGregor and co-researchers from Charing Cross Hospital Medical School in London, have clearly demonstrated that greatly restricting sodium salt intake is both an effective and safe way of treating water retention. By controlling physical symptoms in this way, the patients' level of anxiety about their health may diminish. I have also seen several patients whose marked fluid retention was improved when they avoided certain foods, notably wheat, and this effect appeared not just to be due to its sodium salt content.

Most of the salt in the diets of Westerners used to come from that added in cooking and at the table. However, well over 50 per cent now comes from the salt added to packaged, frozen or tinned foods, so again, it means reading the label. Sodium sulphite and sodium benzoate are used as preservatives, as is ordinary salt (sodium chloride). So beware. Even bread contains significant amounts of salt.

FIBROMYALGIA OR FIBROSITIS

Fibromyalgia is the best of many names that have been used to describe a condition characterised by painful and tender muscles. It has also been termed fibrositis and is a common condition affecting some 12 per cent of patients seen by rheumatologists (specialist doctors who deal with arthritis and muscular complaints). The picture is often one of painful and tender muscles around the shoulder, neck and back. It is more common in women under the age of fifty, and is uncommon in sportspeople and those who are physically fit.

Morning stiffness is a common feature and it can be associated with a poor sleep pattern, headaches, bowel symptoms, anxiety and depression. Again, there is a similarity with chronic fatigue syndrome, just as there is with hyperventilation. A number of abnormalities have been described in people with fibromyalgia, including a disturbed sleep pattern, increased cold sensitivity, subtle changes in muscle chemistry and structure, and minor changes in the immune system.

In the past, sufferers were dismissed as being neurotic but this view is too simplistic, unhelpful and incorrect. For example, Dr Bartels from Oxford and Dr Danneskiold Samasoe from Denmark have shown in biopsy samples from such patients that the muscle fibres of sufferers appear to be constricted by irregular bands. The use of the muscles, therefore, may be inefficient and results in slight tissue damage which sets up inflammation and pain. This produces a picture very similar to that seen in chronic fatigue syndrome where physical activity results in increased pain and fatigue, which discourages the sufferer from exercising. Prolonged rest results in decreasing physical fitness, reduced ability to exercise and a vicious circle. In both fibromyalgia and chronic fatigue syndrome, gentle physical exercise with the acknowledgement that mild fatigue and pain may be experienced along the way is often the best treatment. Additionally, simple painkillers are useful, as is a low dose of the antidepressant amitriptyline which has pain-relieving properties too. This latter may help sleep disturbance if taken at night.

Deficiency of the minerals potassium and magnesium and

vitamin B might also be relevant, as their lack can result in muscle cramps and pain. Relaxation and massage can also be helpful if there are acute muscle spasms. Massage can be made more pleasant by using aromatherapy oils.

RESTLESS LEGS

Believe it or not, the 'restless legs syndrome' has been medically described and is a not infrequent cause of insomnia and it may co-exist with chronic fatigue.

The first clear description was by the Scandinavian neurologist, Professor Ekbom, who reported, 'An unpleasant sensation in the legs, often referred to as "creeping or crawling", usually felt within the calf and shin muscles.' It affects both legs usually, and is most evident at night. The sufferer experiences an irresistible desire to move their legs which can last for several minutes to hours.

Ekbom described this syndrome in association with deficency of the B vitamin folic acid, but it may also occur in people with kidney failure especially if they are anaemic, after bowel surgery, and in diabetics. It seems to occur in some 2 to 5 per cent of the normal population. It has been helped by supplements of folic acid; restriction of tea and coffee; correction of anaemia; and certain drugs, including Clomazepam (a sedative), Levodopa (a drug used for Parkinson's disease), and another drug Carbamazepine. There is also an anecdotal report that a high dose of vitamin E may sometimes be effective. This is one of the few simple distinct causes of a disturbed night's sleep that may usefully respond to a specific type of treatment.

SNORING AND SLEEP APNOEA

The term snoring requires no explanation, but it has recently been defined, for those of us who had any doubt about it, as 'loud upper airway breathing without apnoea or hypoventilation'. There is that word apnoea again. It literally means 'not breathing' and hypoventilation means 'under-breathing'. This also can occur while some people are deeply asleep. Both snoring and under-breathing can, if severe enough, lead to a disturbed night's sleep. They have identifiable and treatable causes and again are worthy of special mention.

They are not entirely innocent problems as those who habitually snore have a significantly increased risk of stroke. Also, snorers tend to be more likely to be sleepy during the day, and this can overlap with a picture of chronic fatigue.

To deal with snorers first, it is more common in men and has a number of causes: narrow nasal air passages, chronic inflammation of the lining of the nose and sinus problems are all factors. Being over-weight, having high blood pressure and consuming excessive amounts of alcohol are also relevant, as is having a relatively large neck size for height.

Many snorers have episodes of sleep apnoea where they stop breathing, or greatly reduce their breathing rate. This is usually noticed by the spouse or bed partner and can cause some alarm as these episodes can last for ten seconds or more. Sleep apnoea itself is related to alcohol, an underactive thyroid gland or other hormonal problems, high blood pressure, use of sedative drugs, and is also associated with diseases of the heart or blood vessels or thickening of the blood.

Often weight reduction, limitation of alcohol consumption and a re-evaluation of drug treatment may improve the quality of these individuals' nights' sleep. Those with heart and lung disease may require treatment of their underlying condition and sometimes oxygen administered continuously at night.

People with milder forms of sleep apnoea syndrome can complain of headache on waking, morning drowsiness, restless sleep, depression, loss of libido, hallucinations at the start of sleep and an increased risk of falling asleep whilst driving. Again there is some overlap with the features of chronic fatigue syndrome.

IRRITABLE BOWEL SYNDROME

Irritable bowel syndrome is very common, occurring according to recent surveys in between 11 and 15 per cent of the normal population. Characteristic features include constipation, diarrhoea or a mixture of the two, abdominal bloating, discomfort and sometimes urgency in going to the toilet. Sometimes pain precedes the desire to open the bowels which is relieved by the passage of a motion. The stools can contain a little mucus or slime, but blood is not usually a feature. Weight loss, severe pain and blood in the stool should all prompt further and detailed investigations, particularly in patients over the age of forty. Irritable bowel syndrome symptoms are very common and are considered to overlap often with post-viral fatigue or chronic fatigue syndromes.

Some psychiatrists have used the presence of these symptoms, together with fatigue, to support a diagnosis of depression. Whilst this might sometimes be justifiable, it should not be allowed to stop the search for possible physical causes or prevent the patient from trying various self-help measures.

In those with constipation and irritable bowel syndrome,

lack of dietary fibre may be important. Supplements of wheat bran are not now thought to be as effective as they once were. Ensuring a good intake of fibre from fruit, vegetables, oats and possibly nuts and seeds, including linseeds, is often helpful and quite soothing on the bowel. For those with diarrhoea, intolerance of milk – lactose – and coffee are possible causes. Unfortunately, however, in patients with both constipation or diarrhoea, intolerance to a wide variety of other foods may occur which may only be detected by following an exclusion diet (see page 254).

Dr John Hunter, a gastro-enterologist at Addenbrooke's Hospital, Cambridge, has investigated many patients with irritable bowel syndrome. From work conducted by him and his colleagues it appears that up to 75 per cent of patients with irritable bowel syndrome can be influenced by diet. The commonest foods for causing bowel upset include wheat, oats, sweetcorn (maize) and other grains, cow's milk and cheese, citrus fruits, tea and coffee, yeast-rich foods, and occasionally many other different types of food.

Some people are known to produce excessive amounts of wind if they eat beans because of their relatively undigestible fibre and carbohydrate content. The undigested fibre may be fermented by the normal or abnormal bacteria that reside in the large bowel (the colon). This may be one of the mechanisms involved in irritable bowel syndrome.

Thus irritable bowel syndrome may be helped by supplements of fibre, following an exclusion diet, and taking drugs to relieve gut spasm or slow down excessively rapid bowel movements. Supplements of healthy bacteria, contained in live yoghurt for instance, may prove to be useful, but this is still uncertain. Occasionally, antibiotics and other measures are required. Stress reduction and the use of hypnosis has also been found to help relieve the symptoms of irritable bowel syndrome. Again, we have a package of physical symptoms with both physical and psychological components contributing to their cause.

LOW BLOOD PRESSURE

It would have been heresy to include low blood pressure as 'a condition' until recently. On continental Europe it has been a popular diagnosis for many years. German doctors apparently have some eighty-five preparations for 'treating' low blood pressure. A number of German medical texts consider that physical and mental fatigue, dizziness, depression and anxiety are all related to low blood pressure (hypotension).

There are a number of rare medical causes, including heart disease, Addison's disease – failure of the adrenal glands – and very rarely, excess activity of the adrenal glands due to a tumour known as phaeochromocytoma. A drop in blood pressure can also occur after eating a meal, particularly in the elderly, and this has been shown to improve with supplements of potassium.

In addition to these known conditions and situations, low blood pressure has recently been found, in a very large survey of men and women in the United Kingdom, to be associated with dizziness and giddiness in men and unexplained tiredness in both men and women. These were surprising and unexpected findings – a rare example of British thinking being brought into line with the EC. The results were published in the *British Medical Journal* at the beginning of 1992. Whether low blood pressure causes these symptoms, or whether other factors relating to physical fitness and personality influence blood pressure and also mental symptoms, is uncertain.

I would favour the latter interpretation. What we are

discovering is that the 'normal population' includes a wide variety of individuals. Those at the extreme, with low blood pressure or high blood pressure, very constipated or with diarrhoea, or those with fatigue, have a complex of physical and mental symptoms which are often associated. They can be interpreted as a 'lack of robustness'. It is unlikely that treatment with any single agent, drug, tonic or vitamin is going to help and one should best consider approaches that combine a number of treatments together.

OBESITY

Is is not clear how relevant obesity is to chronic fatigue syndrome. It is, however, worth considering. Certainly, being over-weight is associated with depression, lack of physical fitness, a lower level of physical exercise and impairment of immune function. It is well known that obesity increases the risk of high blood pressure, heart disease, strokes, gall stones, gout and increases the degree of disability in arthritis.

The abundance of food in Western nations has made it easy for some 30 per cent of adults to become significantly over-weight. Specifically with regard to chronic fatigue syndrome, being over-weight is going to limit the degree to which rehabilitating exercise can take place. Losing weight is therefore important, and a nutritious, high-protein, weight-reducing diet is included in Part 2 (see pages 229–36).

It is recommended if you are over-weight and plan to follow a weight-loss diet for more than four weeks, that you also take a multivitamin supplement which contains zinc too, and if you are a woman who is having periods then one containing iron as well. This is because of the restrictions to your diet and the association of minor abnormalities of immune function with obesity and mild nutrient deficiencies. Indeed, supplementation with these nutrients has been shown to correct minor immune abnormalities within four weeks in obese individuals.

CONCLUSION

As you can see, there are many common minor conditions that overlap with chronic fatigue syndrome. Fortunately, we now know a considerable amount about some of the physical and psychological factors that contribute to these problems. Even if we knew nothing about chronic fatigue syndrome, addressing these problems by standard and accepted means may help to reduce the burden of physical symptoms. This in turn may bring a genuine sense of relief to the sufferer. By lifting their spirits, encouraging them to eat well and take a more positive attitude to their life, and perhaps beginning some physical exercise, a significant and lasting improvement in chronic fatigue can be achieved. In the final analysis, often only the patient him or herself can determine how much of their symptoms are caused by physical factors and how much by emotional and psychological factors.

15

Fatigue and problems of sleep

Disturbance of sleep pattern is accepted as being part of chronic fatigue syndrome. You may be getting less sleep, have difficulty in dropping off or staying asleep and may feel your sleep is unrefreshing or excessive. Similar changes can also occur in depression and this can be misleading. Rather than concentrate on whether changes in sleep pattern are a part of a depressive process or part of chronic fatigue, it is more useful to look at the causes of sleep problems and the practical ways in which they can be tackled.

TOO LITTLE SLEEP – INSOMNIA

This can broadly be divided into two categories: difficulty getting off to sleep and difficulty maintaining sleep. Both are affected by similar factors. A disturbance of sleep pattern with a lack of or unrestful sleep is a recognised feature of chronic fatigue, and it can have a substantial effect on day-time energy levels, drowsiness, concentration, reaction times, mood, perceived stress levels and possibly immunity.

The widespread use of sleeping tablets is an indication of how common this problem is in the general population and how superficially it has often been treated. Approximately one third of the adult population in the United Kingdom experience difficulty falling asleep or a broken night's sleep. So disturbance of sleep is a common enough problem to require addressing in its own right, particularly when fatigue and many related symptoms can accompany it or occur as a result of the prolonged or inappropriate use of the many sedatives used to treat it.

The main factors that influence sleep can be considered under the following headings:

Physical

- Pain from any cause including the muscular and joint aches of chronic fatigue syndromes.
- Any cause of needing to urinate frequently at night, e.g. prostate or bladder problems.
- Fever.
- Chronic heart and lung disease.
- Skin itching.
- Restless legs syndrome (yes, it really does exist).
- Deficiency of B vitamins.

Physiological

- Reduction in sleep requirement with increasing age.
- Shift work or jet-lag.
- Eating late in the evening.
- Exercising late in the evening.

Psychological

- Stress related, e.g. major life changes or pressing problems.

Psychiatric

- Alcoholism.
- Anxiety.
- Depression.
- Mania.

Pharmacological (chemical)

- Caffeine from coffee, tea, cola-based drinks and pain-killers, many of which contain caffeine so read the label carefully.
- Alcohol.
- Side-effects of some drugs.

OVERCOMING INSOMNIA

Treatment obviously should address the underlying causes. Sedatives – which are mainly of the benzodiazepine class of drugs e.g. diazepam and temazepam – are of little long-term value and the manufacturer's recommendation now is that they are only used for a few weeks at a time. They can be useful to help establish a normal sleeping pattern or when lack of sleep is seriously aggravating mental symptoms. A small evening dose of an antidepressant can also be helpful as it may ease any pain.

The use of these drugs should always be combined with

other approaches including dietary change, the use of nutritional supplements and rehabilitation regimes as described below. A more enlightened approach than just handing out the pills is to encourage those with insomnia to practise good sleep 'hygiene'. The recommendations that follow are taken, with a little modification, from those of Dr George Beaumont, a British expert in psychiatry.

Sleep hygiene

- Go to bed at a regular time each night and get up at a regular time each morning. Though this may be difficult at first it will help to establish a regular sleep pattern.
- Make sure that the bedroom is warm, dark, quiet and adequately ventilated but not draughty.
- Wind down in the hour or two before going to bed. Television, videos or involved or stressful conversations may leave you too stimulated to relax easily.
- Reading, listening to music, relaxation exercises or yoga can put you in a more peaceful state of mind.
- Don't eat too late at night. A large meal can take three to four hours to digest fully. This may be particularly relevant for the elderly and those with heart problems.
- Equally don't go to bed feeling hungry. For some a hot milky drink can aid a good night's sleep. If you wake up in the middle of the night a light drink or snack may even help you get back to sleep.
- Establish a routine at bed time – washing or having a warm and relaxing bath, cleaning your teeth, making sure the bedroom is tidy and setting the alarm clock for that rise and shine time.
- Avoid stimulants especially in the evening, e.g. tea, coffee, chocolate-based drinks, excessive alcohol and

nicotine. Women and non-smokers are more sensitive to the effects of caffeine.

* If a small alcoholic drink helps you sleep have one. Many a doctor can testify to the merits of a nightcap to help unwind at the end of a stress-filled day spent prescribing tranquillisers to his patients. Too many drinks, alcoholic or otherwise, will mean that you are more likely to get up at night to pass water, a common cause of a disturbed night's sleep in the elderly.
* Avoid strenuous exercise last thing at night. This is not likely to be a problem for the fatigued.
* If pain is a problem then take a suitable painkiller before retiring. Though most last for only four to six hours there are some long-acting preparations so do ask your doctor about this if appropriate.
* Don't take your worries to bed. You are not likely to solve them in your sleep. It can be helpful to write them down on a piece of paper or to finish off any pressing work rather than to lie awake with thoughts of them running through your mind.
* Avoid prolonged naps during the day. They can interfere with establishing a good natural rhythm of night-time sleep and day-time wakefulness.

DIFFICULTY MAINTAINING SLEEP

This can be a separate problem or accompany difficulty getting off to sleep. The recommendations are the same as those above but particular attention needs to be paid to conditions such as hunger, pain, cold or breathing difficulties. Typically depression can produce early morning waking and may respond to treatment with an antidepressant drug.

TOO MUCH SLEEP

Too much sleep is also a feature of both chronic fatigue states and depression as well as being caused by some physical factors.

If you have a history of depression and find it hard to rally in the mornings you may be surprised to hear that going to bed early and getting up early can improve your mood and general well-being. In fact, a study conducted by Drs Barbara Parry and Thomas Wehr from the National Institute for Mental Health in Bethesda, Maryland, has shown that this is also an effective treatment for those with premenstrual syndrome. They imposed a sleep cycle of 8 p.m. to 2 a.m. on a small group of women with premenstrual depression. There was a significant reduction in depression scores compared with sleeping from 2 a.m. to 8 p.m. It sounds a little drastic but the overall message is, 'Don't stay in bed too long'.

In conclusion some people with chronic fatigue, without a major physical component, who have a slow start in the morning after a long unrefreshing night's sleep would do well to try going to bed early, getting up early and perhaps either going for a short walk or doing something constructive and pleasant on rising. Getting the day off to a good start is one of the simple self-help measures worth practising.

PART 2

The treatment of fatigue

16

Chronic fatigue – the treatment plan

The evidence from numerous publications in medical journals indicates that there are many effective treatments for chronic fatigue. By now you should have some idea which of them is appropriate for you but you may wish to discuss this with your doctor before proceeding further.

The concept of the treatment plan is to try and improve your physical and psychological health as much as possible. There is little point differentiating between the two as they are so closely linked. Physical health can be influenced by the type of diet you eat, the balance of nutrients in your diet, how much sleep you have and your physical activity level. All these things, together with lifestyle, personal, psychological and social factors also influence mental health.

The treatment programme is broken up into different sections which deal with different aspects of health.

THE TREATMENT PLAN

The treatment plan may consist of any combination of the following which can be tailored to your specific condition and needs:

- Dietary treatments. This consists of essentially two types of diet: either a very nutritious diet or an exclusion diet.
- Lifestyle changes: strategies for reducing stress and coping with fatigue.
- The use of gentle exercise to aid recovery.
- Pills and potions: nutritional supplements and drugs that can help fatigue.
- Complementary treatments such as osteopathy, acupuncture and herbal medicine that can provide some benefit.
- Getting a good night's sleep (covered in Chapter 15).

It is difficult if not impossible to know at the outset which of these, or more probably which combination of these, is right for any one individual. Having read through Part 1 you may well have an idea as to which aspects of your life or healthcare need addressing. By looking at all of the following chapters you should be able to assess which areas are more important for you and also in which ones it is actually feasible for you to follow some of the recommendations that are given.

For example, if you are experiencing only mild fatigue that has not been severe enough to affect your lifestyle then it would be perfectly reasonable to make various changes to your diet, perhaps try certain types of nutritional supplements and some gentle physical exercise without recourse to further advice from your doctor.

If, however, you have been seeing your own family practitioner or a specialist because the fatigue has been severe, then you should check with your doctor again before embarking upon these approaches. Indeed he may be able to offer you further advice about dietary treatment or refer you on to a dietary specialist. Additionally, he may be able to prescribe certain nutritional supplements for you and perhaps carry out some tests to assess which ones would be the most appropriate.

If your fatigue continues to be severe or you have a fever with worsening physical symptoms, then your doctor should be looking for any undiagnosed physical illness.

17

A very nutritious diet

There are two main dietary options for you to follow, depending on your requirements. This chapter deals with the first option.

A VERY NUTRITIOUS DIET FOR FATIGUE

The concept of this diet is that it is rich in essential vitamins, minerals and protein, and low or devoid of foods that are high in calories but low in nutrients. It is similar to many convalescent diets from the last one hundred years or so. There are also a variety of options for you to choose from depending upon your needs:

- Weight – under-weight or over-weight.
- Vegetarian or vegan.
- Migraine headaches.
- Fluid retention.
- Irritable bowel syndrome.
- Premenstrual syndrome.
- Allergies.

You need to decide which type of diet would best fit your fatigue symptoms. If you are over-weight, then you need to follow a basic diet with the recommendations for those who need to lose weight. Additionally, if you are a vegetarian then you need to follow that section, and if you also have migraine headaches then check the other dietary advice and the list of foods that should be avoided in that part too. It is possible to combine options in this way. It, however, is not very feasible to combine more than two options out of the migraine, fluid retention, irritable bowel syndrome, pre-menstrual syndrome and allergies sections. It is not that the advice would conflict, but it would start to become very complicated. Therefore you would probably be better advised to move on to the next chapter – Exclusion Diets (page 254).

The dietary treatments in this chapter would need to be followed for several weeks or possibly two or three months before any improvement could be anticipated. For example, it could take as long as three months of eating a very healthy diet to correct mild nutritional deficiencies of, say, iron or B vitamins. Similarly, if you are over-weight it could take anything from six weeks to six months to bring your weight down to a satisfactory level.

The recommendations for vegetarians would need to be followed long term as might those recommendations given for fluid retention and allergies. For migraine, irritable bowel syndrome and premenstrual syndrome, you may have to try some dietary experimentation. By this I mean that if there is improvement in the first stages of the diet – within the first four to eight weeks – it would become necessary to try reintroducing foods in a controlled manner to determine which might be contributing to these problems and/or your fatigue. This concept is explored further in Chapter 18, Exclusion Diets, beginning on page 254.

What are the main features of the 'Very Nutritious Diet'?

- It's high in protein, vitamins and minerals.
- It's very pleasant. Pleasure in its own right improves mood and helps recovery.
- It's easy to follow.

In order to stick to the recommendations you will need to go shopping at least twice a week, or more frequently if you do not have a fridge or freezer.

General recommendations

- *Eat regularly.* Have three meals a day: breakfast, lunch and supper, and snacks in between. Details about nutritious snacks can be found on page 222. Each meal should contain some protein-rich foods, see below.
- Sugar, sweet foods and refined carbohydrates should be kept to a minimum. Sugar (sucrose) and foods rich in sugar are high in calories and low in essential vitamins and minerals. It is perfectly all right to have small amounts of sugar in foods such as a little jam, marmalade and the occasional biscuit or cake, if these are not excluded for other reasons. Ice cream is also allowed in modest quantities as its dairy content makes it moderately nutritious. However, it is important to limit your intake of sweets, chocolate, sugar added to tea and coffee, soft drinks, and to avoid large quantities of cakes, biscuits, puddings and pies. Small amounts of honey are also allowed.
- Have a regular daily intake of fresh fruit. You should have at least three pieces of fresh fruit per day. Fruit contains fruit sugar (fructose) which does not have the same effect on the metabolism as ordinary sugar (sucrose).

- Have a regular daily intake of fresh vegetables, especially green ones. Vegetables are rich in the vitamins and minerals that are most commonly found to be lacking in many ill or elderly people.

  If you only go shopping once or twice a week, then keep the green vegetables in a cool place, or even in the bottom of the fridge. Frozen vegetables are acceptable and frozen peas are a convenient, cheap and nutritious food.

- Have a good daily intake of protein-rich foods (vegetarians see vegetarian section on page 236). It is recommended that you have meat, fish or poultry at least once a day. A good portion size is about 160 grams (6 oz) pre-cooked weight, but you may need more if you are of a large build and physically active. Other protein-rich foods with approximate weekly consumption guides are: eggs (three to six per week); beans or peas (two to four portions per week); milk (two to seven pints per week); cheese (100 to 300 grams/4 to 12 oz per week); and nuts or seeds (optional). Smaller amounts of protein are found in potatoes, rice, sweetcorn (maize) and bread. Have a good amount of two of these every day.

- Avoid bran, bran-containing cereals and large amounts of wholemeal bread. Bran is high in phytic acid which blocks the absorption of calcium, magnesium, zinc and iron. Some people, particularly those with digestive problems, may find that it aggravates this problem. Replace bran-containing cereals with either oats, corn or rice-based cereals. These latter two, if they are fortified with vitamins and iron, are particularly suitable. Their fibre content, however, is not very high but you can increase this by adding fruit, nuts or seeds to them.

- Bread intake should be limited to two to four slices per day. The fibre from fruit and vegetables is now considered in some ways to be healthier than that derived from cereal products. For other reasons, including food allergy or intolerance, it may be prudent to limit your intake of wheat. You can have white bread or whole-meal, whichever suits you better.

- Alcohol consumption should be very moderate. Many patients with severe fatigue are better off not having any alcohol at all. The current safe recommendations for men are up to three units per day, and women two units a day (one unit = half a pint normal strength beer or lager = one measure of spirits = 1 glass of wine = one small measure of Vermouth or sherry). Women who are pregnant, trying to get pregnant, and men and women with liver disease or who have abnormal liver function tests should not consume alcohol.

- Eat nutritious snacks. As well as having three meals a day, you should have regular and nutritious snacks. This will ensure a good nutrient intake and will prevent excessive swings in blood sugar or changes in metabolism as a result of eating infrequently. Additionally, large meals may not be digested easily in some unwell or elderly patients.

  Nutritious snacks include: a piece of fruit; bread or a rice cake with a nut spread; a low-fat yoghurt; nuts and dried fruit; nuts and fresh fruit; a small piece of cheese; and fruit or raw vegetables and dips.

  If it is particularly important for you to eat regularly, make sure that you have plenty of suitable and pleasant snack foods at home, at work, in the car or in your bag. This is one of the best ways of avoiding bingeing or relying upon non-nutritious snacks such as chocolate bars, sweets, cakes, etc.

- Have a reasonable intake of dairy products. A good average is half to one pint of milk per day, and 100 to

225 grams (4 to 8 oz) of cheese per week. Those who are over-weight will need to have low-fat versions. Milk can be added to tea and coffee.

- Tea and coffee consumption should not be excessive. Limit tea to two cups a day and coffee to two cups a day. They are perhaps best avoided if insomnia or anxiety are a problem, and vegetarian women may need to make further limitations – see below.

- Enjoy your food and eat in company. It has been observed repeatedly that the nutrient intake of those who live alone is not as good as those who live with others or share their meals with them. Eating is potentially a great pleasure and one that you can experience every day. If you do live alone, then arrange to visit friends or invite them round to you so that you can share the pleasure of having a good meal together.

Very nutritious diet – sample menus

Here are some sample menus for you to make a start with:

Breakfast 1

2 poached eggs
grilled tomatoes
mushrooms
2 slices of wholemeal or white toast with sunflower spread
    or butter and marmalade
a glass of orange juice

Breakfast 2

muesli
chopped fruit
crumbled pecan nuts with milk or live yoghurt
2 slices of wholemeal or white toast with peanut butter
herbal tea or coffee substitute

Breakfast 3

1 egg and cheese omelette
2 slices of wholemeal or white toast with sunflower spread
   or butter and lemon curd or jam
a glass of fruit juice or herbal tea

Mid-morning snacks

Choose between:
fruit, nuts and seeds
cheese and biscuits
fruit yoghurt

Lunch 1

sardines, tuna, mackerel or salmon
potato salad
mixed green salad
fresh fruit
herbal tea

Lunch 2

grilled chicken
brown rice and vegetable salad
coleslaw and mixed salad

a glass of orange juice

Lunch 3

jacket potato with baked beans and melted cheese
mixed green salad with oil dressing
a glass of apple juice

Mid-afternoon snacks

toast and peanut butter
flapjack and herbal tea
any of the morning snacks

Dinner 1

prawn and vegetable stir fry
egg fried rice
fruit and oat flapjacks

Dinner 2

2 lamb chops grilled or good-sized steak
baked potato
fresh greens and peas
stuffed baked apples or fruit crumble

Dinner 3

chicken and cashew nut curry
pilau rice
curried mixed vegetables
apple and cinnamon pancakes with whipped cream

UNDER-WEIGHT

If you have lost a lot of weight due to your illness or if you have been chronically under-weight, then you should eat as healthily as possible to improve your weight. To achieve this, you may want to follow some of the additional recommendations:

General recommendations

- Always *eat regularly* and *never miss* meals. Missing a meal is missing an opportunity to have an improved nutrient intake, so take particular care with this.
- Eat regular, *nutritious* snacks. Many people who have lost weight cannot eat large meals, and so the best advice for them is to eat little and often. Nutritious and high-calorie snack foods include bananas, avocado pears, cheese, full-fat milk and milk-shakes, nuts and seeds, and nut spreads such as peanut or almond which can be spread on to bread or rice cakes. Some of these can be combined with fruit.
- Have plenty of dairy products. Use liberal amounts of cheese, milk, cream and ice cream. Add milk or cream to sauces, have vegetables with melted cheese or a cheese sauce, and have fruit salad as a dessert with cream or ice cream. These are all good ways of improving your calorie, protein and nutrient intake. If you are intolerant to cow's milk dairy products use soya milk instead. Calcium-fortified soya milk is now available in many supermarkets.
- Small amounts of chocolate and sweet foods are allowable. They are best taken at the end of a meal so as not to interfere with your appetite.
- Try having a snack or warm milky drink at night. Again,

some people find that this is a convenient way of increasing their nutrient intake.

- Allow yourself some fried foods! Use a good quality vegetable oil: corn, sunflower, safflower or rapeseed oil. Fresh-made, home-cooked, thick-cut chips are not only delicious, but still contain a reasonable amount of vitamin C.

- Make modest use of oil-rich salad dressings. Olive oil or other fine oils, e.g. walnut, almond or grapeseed oil, make excellent salad dressings either on their own or mixed with vinegar and herbs. There are many such prepared dressings available in supermarkets and delicatessens. They will help you to keep your calorie intake up.

- You can have sugar-containing breakfast cereals in moderation. You can eat the frosted or sugared versions of fortified corn, rice and some wheat cereals available, or alternatively, you can add one or two teaspoons of sugar to a non-sugared version. Do not, however, consume them to excess (and preferably don't feed them to children).

- Use liquid meals if eating is difficult. For some, especially the very ill and elderly, eating adequately is difficult. A convenient and nutritious source of nutrients are various liquid feeds that can be made up with milk or water. These can be used as a snack or as a replacement meal. Follow the manufacturer's guidelines. Most are fortified with good amounts of vitamins and minerals to help ensure nutrient adequacy. Homemade soups with added milk or cream are also easy to eat and nutritious.

Under-weight diet – sample menus

Breakfast 1

2 eggs cooked any way – even fried
grilled bacon and mushrooms or tomatoes
1 or 2 slices of toast with marmalade
a glass of orange juice or herbal tea

Breakfast 2

bowl of muesli or fortified cereal (e.g. corn flakes or rice
    crispies) with extra nuts e.g. almonds, walnuts or pecans,
    and stewed fruit
1 or 2 slices of white or wholemeal toast with peanut butter,
    jam or marmalade
piece of fruit e.g. banana
a glass of fruit juice

Mid-morning snacks

fresh fruit, avocados, dates, dried fruit
yoghurt, (not low-fat), cheese, cold meat
milk, milk-shakes, fruit juice
cup of herbal tea or very weak ordinary tea with a teaspoon
    of honey or sugar

Lunch 1

baked potato with a filling, such as tuna in oil with chopped
    onions or peppers and mayonnaise, cheese, baked beans,
    sweet corn and butter or margarine
a glass of juice
yoghurt (not low-fat), piece of fruit, bread and jam

Lunch 2

bowl of soup with added cream or cheese
2 pieces of bread – white or wholemeal and butter or
    margarine
piece of fruit

Mid-afternoon snacks

As before, or occasional scones and low-sugar jam

Dinner 1

roast meat – beef, pork, lamb, etc.
roast potatoes and two or more other vegetables
fruit salad and ice cream

Dinner 2

fish baked or poached
mashed potatoes with added milk/cream/cheese
two or more other vegetables
rice pudding or pancakes with stewed fruit and cream or
    apple pie and ice cream

Any of the suggested menus in the basic Very Nutritious Diet
can also be used in part or in whole.

OVER-WEIGHT

Remember that being over-weight can contribute to fatigue
by having an adverse effect on your immune function,
physical fitness, mood, your own self-esteem and morale.

General recommendations

- Use low-calorie versions of dairy products. Use skimmed or semi-skimmed milk (half to one pint a day) and low-fat cheeses limited to no more than 150 grams (6 oz) per week.

- Avoid sugar (sucrose), glucose, sweets, cakes, biscuits, chocolate, puddings *completely*. Allow yourself small amounts of reduced-sugar jams and marmalade, and if your weight loss is satisfactory, you might perhaps break the diet once or twice a week, allowing yourself a small amount of a favourite dessert, e.g. reduced-calorie ice cream.

- Use oils and fat spreads sparingly. There are low-calorie, polyunsaturated fat spreads, and limit yourself to one teaspoon of these per day. Allow yourself one teaspoon of ordinary oil for use either in salad dressing or for frying. Stir fry meals require little oil and can be very nutritious.

- Limit fruit to three pieces per day. A large banana counts as two units of fruit. Only have fruit juices occasionally as they provide calories without the fibre.

- Avoid soft drinks which contain several hundred calories. Have low-calorie versions instead, but again limit these to half to one can per day. It is all too easy to consume large quantities of these. Consuming them regularly will help maintain a taste for sweet foods. Their high phosphate content may, if consumed to excess, interfere with the absorption of calcium and magnesium.

- Trim all visible fat from meat and poultry before cooking. Do not eat chicken or fish skins. Cook meat, fish and chicken by grilling or baking (broiling). Do not fry them.

- Use low-fat salad dressings and sauces. For instance, instead of making sauces with cream, you can use tinned tomatoes with herbs.
- Eat large amounts of salad and green vegetables. These are very nutritious and low in calories. You can add low-fat mayonnaise or salad dressing to them, allowing yourself twenty to thirty calories of these per day. Follow the calorie guide given on the container.
- Potatoes can be eaten. Allow yourself one 150 gram (6 oz) potato per day, i.e. slightly smaller than the size of your fist.
- Allow yourself only two slices of bread per day. It is very easy to eat more than this, and though bread is not high in calories, it is easy to add butter or margarine and sugar-containing spreads which then greatly increase its calorie content.
- Eat regularly and have *small* snacks between meals. This will help keep your appetite down and your weight loss will be slightly better if the calorie load is spread evenly throughout the day, rather than having one or two large meals per day.
- You may use convenience low-calorie meals. They are particularly useful if you are working or you are limited as to what you can do in the kitchen. Most provide around 300 calories and have a modest protein and nutrient intake. Their nutrient intake cannot be fully relied upon, however, and if you eat them regularly, it is prudent to have a multivitamin supplement too. You can gain many of the nutrients that are low in these meals, such as iron and B vitamins, by having an additional portion of salad or green vegetables. These provide few calories, but make up for some of the absent essential nutrients. Try not to have convenience low-calorie meals more than three or four times per week.

- Choose an unsugared breakfast cereal allowing yourself 30 to 50 grams (1 to 1½ oz) for a breakfast portion. Cornflakes, fortified corn and rice breakfast cereals are quite nutritious and not high in calories, particularly if taken with skimmed milk.

This is just an outline of some of the dietary recommendations you will need to follow to help lose weight. Many men and women find it helpful to join a local slimming club or class. Some of these are organised through a doctor's surgery, hospital, local slimming club representative, health club or other private institution. The success you'll have at such slimming clubs is largely dependent upon your regular attendance and the support you receive from the course organiser and fellow dieters. A book or diet sheet is no substitute for this degree of support, so seek it out if you need it.

Here are some sample menus for you to make a start with:

Weight-loss diet – sample menus

Breakfast 1

	calories
2 poached eggs	160
2 grilled tomatoes	16
115 grams (4 oz) poached mushrooms	14
2 slices of slimmer's bread	80
1 teaspoon low-calorie margarine	25
2 teaspoons low-calorie jam	20
cup of black decaffeinated tea	0
Total calories	315

Breakfast 2

1 portion of chopped fruit	50
55 grams (2 oz) Jordan's special muesli	95
85 ml (3 fl oz) skimmed milk	28
1 slice of wholemeal toast	70
1 teaspoon low-calorie margarine	25
1 teaspoon low-calorie jam	10
cup of black decaffeinated coffee	0

Total calories   278

Breakfast 3

1 egg and cheese omelette (15 grams or $\frac{1}{2}$ oz)	137
1 slice of slimmer's toast or 2 rice cakes	56
1 teaspoon low-calorie spread	25
2 teaspoons low-calorie jam	20
cup of black decaffeinated tea or coffee	0

Total calories   238

Mid-morning snacks

100 grams ($3\frac{1}{2}$ oz) low-fat yoghurt	40
one grated apple	50
or	
1 portion of fruit (except bananas which are approx double calories of other fruits)	50
or	
115 grams (4 oz) raw carrot	26
170 grams (6 oz) sticks celery	12

Lunch 1

140 grams (5 oz) sardines in tomato sauce, tinned	250
115 grams (4 oz) potato salad	125
225 grams (8 oz) mixed green salad	32
cup of herb tea without milk	0
Total calories	407

Lunch 2

115 gram (4 oz) chicken drumstick, grilled	84
225 gram (8 oz) portion of mixed green salad	32
172 gram (6 oz) portion of coleslaw	40
172 gram (6 oz) brown rice and vegetable salad	55
115 millilitre (14 fl oz) orange juice	50
Total calories	261

Lunch 3

172 gram (6 oz) jacket potato	144
2 teaspoons low-calorie margarine	50
225 grams (8 oz) low-calorie baked beans	122
225 grams (8 oz) mixed green salad	32
115 grams (4 oz) glass apple juice	50
Total calories	398

Mid-afternoon snacks

2 rice cakes with 2 teaspoons low-calorie jam	
cup of decaffeinated tea with milk	81

or
30 grams (1 oz) dried apricots   51
or
2 tablespoons of raisins and 15 grams ($\frac{1}{2}$oz) of
   unsalted peanuts   90

Dinner 1

280 grams (10 oz) prawn and vegetable stir fry   225
55 grams (2 oz) brown rice   66
   mixed with 30 grams (1 oz) hazelnuts   95
1 slice of oat flapjack   115
                                      ———

Total calories   501

Dinner 2

115 grams (4 oz) lamb chop, grilled   222
115 grams (4 oz) boiled potatoes   90
115 grams (4 oz) cabbage   10
115 grams (4 oz) sweetcorn   86
Baked apple and 55 grams (2 oz) low-calorie
   ice cream   140
                                      ———

Total calories   548

Dinner 3

medium serving of vegetable curry   185
55 grams (2 oz) brown rice   66
2 pancakes with lemon and sugar   150
                                      ———

Total calories   401

N.B. The calorific values given are approximate, and will vary from product to product.

VEGETARIANS

Vegetarian diets can be extremely healthy, but are not necessarily so. A good vegetarian diet can be rich in all essential nutrients and protein. They may provide particularly good amounts of magnesium and B vitamins. However, some foods may be relatively low in protein and iron, and thus care has to be taken.

General recommendations

- Avoid too much sugar and refined foods. Large intakes of sugar (sucrose), sweets, cakes, biscuits and so forth, simply displace more nutritious foods from the diet. Allow yourself some, but do not consume them to excess. A 'junk food', poorly balanced vegetarian diet can be one of the worst diets eaten. Teenage girls and women in their early twenties are particularly prone to eating this type of diet.
- Have a good intake of protein-rich foods. This includes nuts, seeds, peas, beans, lentils, whole grains, eggs, dairy products, sweetcorn (maize) and to a lesser extent, potatoes and rice. Weekly recommendations for these foods are as follows:

Eggs three to seven per week, unless you are known to have a very high blood cholesterol.
Milk/yoghurt/cream up to a pint per day.
Cheese 225–450 grams (8 to 16 oz) per week.
Beans any type excluding green beans: 335–450 grams

(12 to 16 oz) (cooked weight) per week (two to four portions).

Frozen peas 225–450 grams (8 to 12 oz) per week (two to three portions).

Nuts and seeds any type: 450 grams (8 oz) per week.

Potatoes three to four portions per week.

Corn as sweetcorn or cornflakes: two to seven portions per week.

Wholemeal bread three to six slices per day (unless to be avoided).

Other whole grain cereals e.g. wholemeal pasta, cracked wheat, barley and rye: two to three portions per week.

Soya-based proteins e.g. textured vegetable protein (TVP): two to three portions per week.

Other protein sources e.g. Quinoa or Quorn: two to three portions per week.

The figures quoted are all moderately high goals, and it is assumed that the average vegetarian will be consuming only about two-thirds of these foods during the course of the average week. It is important that a good variety of different foods is achieved. In this way, the intake of essential amino acids, which are derived from protein-rich foods, will be adequate. Each individual vegetable-derived food does not contain the full complement of essential amino acids, but these can easily be obtained by ensuring an adequate mix and balance of these vegetable foods, or combining them with dairy products and eggs.

• Certain combinations of vegetarian protein-rich foods will help to ensure an adequate supply of essential amino acids. Each vegetable-derived food contains some, but not all, of the essential amino acids. Therefore, to ensure you are getting enough in your diet, a good balance of these vegetable proteins needs to be achieved.

Combinations that provide good balances of proteins within a meal are:

> Rice with beans or sesame seeds or cheese.
> Wheat with – beans
> – mixed nuts + milk
> – sesame seeds and soya beans.
> Corn with beans.
> Mixed nuts with sunflower seeds.

Adding dairy products – milk or cheese, and eggs – to any vegetable protein will improve the protein content of the meal, and provide a better balance of the essential amino acids. Amino acids are important for health, especially muscle function and immune system function. Deficiency of individual amino acids is exceptionally rare.

- Keep intakes of tea and coffee to a minimum. The tannin content of tea greatly inhibits absorption of iron from non-meat protein sources. This recommendation is particularly relevant for women who are menstruating. Having fruit or fresh vegetables which contain vitamin C enhances iron absorption, and these should form a good part of all vegetarians' diets anyway. The use of iron-fortified breakfast cereals is a convenient way of improving iron intake, especially if they are consumed with fruit or fruit juice.

- Avoid bran. Again, bran, because of its phytic acid content, inhibits the absorption of iron as well as calcium, magnesium and zinc. The health benefits of wheatbran in particular have been greatly over-rated and it is best avoided. Oats, rice and soya bran may be less harmful in this respect, but it is still better to obtain your fibre from fruit, vegetables, beans and seeds.

- Special situations. If you are a vegetarian or a vegan and have lost a considerable amount of weight recently you will require expert advice from a dietician or doctor. Also, life-long vegans require careful assessment if they are troubled by fatigue as they may be at particular risk of vitamin B12 deficiency. Vegetarians and vegans who are pregnant also need dietary advice from a qualified dietician.

Vegetarian diet – sample menus

Here are some sample menus for you to make a start with:

Breakfast 1

muesli with chopped banana and milk
toast and marmalade
herbal tea or fresh fruit juice
a glass of fresh orange juice

Breakfast 2

scrambled eggs and tomatoes on toast
herbal tea or coffee substitute

Breakfast 3

fresh fruit salad with yoghurt
toast and peanut butter
herbal tea or fresh fruit juice

Mid-morning snacks

fruit, nuts and seeds
cheese and biscuits
fruit yoghurt

Lunch 1

jacket potato with cheese
green salad sprinkled with sesame seeds or nuts
fresh fruit

Lunch 2

vegetable soup
French bread with mixed bean salad
nuts and raisins

Lunch 3

raw vegetables and corn chips with humous dip
live fruit yoghurt

Mid-afternoon snacks

cream tea
toast and peanut butter
flapjack

Dinner 1

nut loaf
green vegetables, parsnips and carrots
buckwheat, apple and cinnamon pancakes

Dinner 2

stir fry vegetables and nuts
egg fried rice
flapjacks

Dinner 3

vegetable and nut curry (cashew or peanut or substitute with
Quorn or TVP chunks)
rice and chapati
fresh fruit compote

The next few sections concentrate on different options for
tackling other associated complaints that you might be
troubled by. They include migraine headaches, fluid retention, irritable bowel syndrome, premenstrual syndrome and
allergies.

MIGRAINE HEADACHES

Migraine headaches can be triggered by emotional or
physical stress, lack of sleep, food allergies or intolerances,
missing meals, withdrawal of tea or coffee, or they can be
related to a woman's menstrual cycle, and very occasionally
be caused by associated medical problems.

Dietary triggers have been well documented. Certain
foods are rich in naturally occurring chemicals called
amines. Some of these affect the blood vessels and are
termed 'vaso-active amines' (literally, amine chemicals that
react with blood vessels). There is now evidence that some
people with migraine are particularly susceptible to these
naturally occurring chemicals, and may have a reduced
ability to break down and detoxify these and other related
compounds.

It is recommended that if you have migraine you should
avoid, or severely limit, intake of the following foods:

- Cheese – all types.
- Chocolate, tea, coffee and cola-based drinks.

- Painkillers containing caffeine.
- Alcoholic beverages.
- Yeast extracts.
- Meat extracts – salami, pepperami and other similar sausages.
- Monosodium glutamate (often shortened to MSG on food labels).

Additionally, some people with migraine headaches may also be intolerant of certain fruits including bananas, plums, oranges, pineapples, tomatoes and avocados, as well as some vegetables, especially broad beans. This is rare though. Very, very occasionally, migraine headaches are precipitated by any intake of protein which can be caused by a metabolic problem (ornithine carbamoyl transferase deficiency). If this is the case, specialist neurological and metabolic assessment is required.

In addition to the foods listed above, it has become increasingly recognised that some migraine headaches are precipitated by other foods including cow's milk and cow's milk-related products, and wheat, oats, barley and rye, perhaps because of their gluten content.

If migraine headaches do not improve with the avoidance of the first group of foods above, you may need to consider avoiding cow's milk and the gluten-containing cereals.

What do to if you get a migraine attack

The acute attack is best treated by:

- Rest, usually going to bed.
- Early treatment with ordinary painkillers (not containing caffeine). Anti-sickness medicines may also be required if nausea and vomiting become a problem.

- Occasionally, you may benefit from breathing in exhaled air by using a paper bag early in an attack. This increases the level of carbon dioxide in the blood which may stop the headache developing.
- Taking sodium bicarbonate may similarly load the system with extra carbon dioxide and stop the headache developing.

Once developed, migraine headaches often have to run their own course, and can only be relieved with stronger pain-killers.

Preventing migraine headaches can be achieved by following the dietary recommendations above, but also may be helped by taking a variety of drugs on a regular basis – your doctor will be able to advise you. Feverfew, it is has been recorded, is also of benefit. This herb is now available in tablet form from health shops. There is also some scientific foundation to the traditional Chinese remedy of ginger which can be taken as crystallised ginger or as a ginger preserve on a daily basis.

FLUID RETENTION

Fluid retention, including premenstrual water retention, can again be influenced by dietary factors. They include:

- Limitation of sodium (salt) intake.
- Restriction of sucrose (sugar) and refined carbohydrates.
- Avoidance of foods to which an allergic or intolerant reaction may be experienced.

By far the most important factor is restriction of sodium intake. This should now really replace any use of diuretics, except those that are used very occasionally or in the short term. Remember that nowadays most of the sodium in our diets comes not from salt added at the table or used in cooking, but salt that is found in prepared foods.

The advice is:

- Do not add salt to cooking.
- Do not add salt at the table.
- Avoid all salty foods. You will have to read the labels and watch out for all sodium containing additives. The main salty foods are salted savoury snacks, e.g. peanuts, potato crisps; salted meats, e.g. ham, smoked meat, smoked fish; many tinned foods, including tinned vegetables, tinned meats and fish; many packaged foods, especially those containing sauces; some frozen foods; many sweet biscuits and cakes, to which salt is also added.

  Many foods contain preservatives and flavour enhancers, which are sodium based. These include sodium sulphite, metabisulphite, sodium benzoate and monosodium glutamate. These may be found not only in savoury foods, but also in sweet drinks, e.g. squash and fizzy drinks. By law, almost all developed countries demand that lists of ingredients are given on the food product, including whether salt and additives are used. Read the label carefully.

  Other common foods that also contain significant amounts of sodium include cheese, bread, crackers and prepared foods that contain cheese, wheat or breadcrumbs. The sodium content may not always be stated in these cases.
- Be aware that some medicines may be high in sodium, especially indigestion and anti-acid preparations.

Unfortunately, it is sometimes necessary to restrict sodium intake severely in order to control fluid retention. Such diets can be difficult and tedious. It is usually useful to obtain further advice on sodium-rich foods, and many helpful books are available in book and health food shops or sheets may be obtained from dieticians. For the technically minded, sodium intake may have to be restricted to 50 millimols of sodium per day, and you can calculate this intake from the information given in such books and lists.

Usually, when beginning a low sodium diet, food tastes bland. However, do persevere as your taste will adjust after six to eight weeks.

Salt substitutes can be used, but only sparingly. They are high in potassium, and potassium accumulation could occur in the elderly, those with kidney problems, those taking diuretics (water tablets) or anti-arthritis drugs. Use herbs and spices to help improve the flavour of food.

In addition to cutting down on sodium salt, limiting intake of sugar (sucrose) may also be helpful. Some people appear to retain more sodium when eating diets high in sugar and other sweet foods. Occasionally, true food allergy or intolerance contributes to fluid retention.

IRRITABLE BOWEL SYNDROME

Irritable bowel syndrome is a common disorder, and there are different dietary and other recommendations depending upon the pattern of symptoms. The commonest symptoms are abdominal bloating, discomfort and pain in association with diarrhoea, constipation, or a mixture of diarrhoea and constipation.

Often, it is the level of pain the person experiences that determines whether or not they seek advice about their problem. Many people just put up with constipation or episodes of diarrhoea. Mild fatigue, indigestion and other symptoms often accompany these lower bowel problems.

If you have constipation

- Eat a diet high in fruit and vegetables.
- Avoid tea. This can aggravate constipation in some people.
- Have a little coffee or another hot drink especially early in the morning as they can help to stimulate the large bowel into action.
- Develop a routine, as opening your bowels at a regular time each day is often easier.
- Try a fibre supplement (preferably not wheat or ordinary bran). Use coarse oats or ispaghula as they retain a lot of water in the stool. Many pharmacy preparations contain ispaghula which is the husk of a tropical plant. Linseeds are also very useful and can be added to your breakfast cereal. Look out for Linusit Gold which is available at most health food shops.
- Take some magnesium supplements which can act as a laxative. Sometimes they also help muscle symptoms and fatigue. Almost any form of magnesium may act as a laxative. Epsom salts, magnesium sulphate, can be a bit dramatic in its effect and the more comfortable types to take are magnesium oxide, or one of the more specialised supplements – magnesium gluconate, citrate or chelate. A suitable daily dosage is usually 300 milligrams per day for an adult, and some people may need to take up to 600 milligrams per day before a laxative effect is experienced. If you are very deficient in magnesium, much of the magnesium may be absorbed. However, if you need to take doses of more than 600 milligrams of

magnesium a day on a regular basis you should first check with your doctor. High doses can cause problems in older patients and those with kidney disease.
- Try some other laxatives. It is best to take advice from your doctor or pharmacist about this especially if you need them on a regular basis. Senokot, which is contained in many herbal laxative preparations, can damage the bowel if taken regularly over many years. It is all right to take it occasionally.

It may be useful to combine a high-fibre diet with a fibre supplement and a modest supplement of magnesium. You may need to try several different types of fibre supplement before you find one that suits your bowels best and that may even be wheatbran. Use your own judgement but don't be afraid to try different approaches until you find the one that suits you.

If you have diarrhoea

- Avoid coffee as it can increase the rate at which food moves through the bowel.
- Avoid spicy foods.
- Avoid any foods that you know upset you.
- If you have associated wind, try avoiding onion, garlic, leeks, beans, peas, lentils, cabbage, cauliflower and broccoli. These frequently aggravate wind in some people but they are all healthy, nutritious vegetables.
- Try eating live yoghurt. There is some evidence that irritable bowel syndrome is in part due to a disturbance in the type of bacteria in the large bowel. This might be helped by taking live yoghurt, but it is a rather hit and miss method.

These measures, however, may not be enough, particularly if your symptoms are severe and if you have alternating diarrhoea and constipation. It is now well known that many patients with irritable bowel syndrome have intolerance to specific foods. Wheat, other grains, dairy products, citrus fruit and yeast-rich foods seem particularly likely to aggravate the symptoms of irritable bowel syndrome.

Stress is also important. Relaxation therapies can help a lot with this. If pain is particularly a problem then drugs that stop the spasm may be useful. Peppermint also has a relaxing effect on the gut and there are some specialised preparations for irritable bowel syndrome that contain it. Ask your doctor.

If your symptoms do not respond to the above measures, then following a partial exclusion diet (see page 255) may be helpful.

PREMENSTRUAL SYNDROME

Fatigue may co-exist with premenstrual syndrome. Indeed, it has been known for over fifty years that fatigue can occur in many healthy women before their period. Some of this may be physiological – due to natural fluctuations in hormone levels and metabolism. If the fatigue is severe, and in particular if it is associated with mood swings, irritability, breast tenderness and fluid retention, then additional dietary measures may be important. The diet can be combined with supplements of magnesium, together with vitamin B6 and multivitamins (see page 157). If premenstrual breast tenderness is a particular problem, supplements of evening primrose oil can also be taken. Exercise is also of proven benefit in PMS.

General recommendations

- Take care to follow the recommendations for a nutritious diet. This is very important.
- If over- or under-weight, follow those recommendations too. Adjusting your weight may make a big difference to your hormone metabolism.
- If premenstrual breast tenderness is a problem, restrict your intake of foods rich in saturated (animal) fats and ensure you have a good intake of proteins from vegetable and animal sources. This means using low-fat dairy products; using good quality vegetable oils – sunflower, safflower, corn or rapeseed oil – and only in small quantities; using polyunsaturate-rich margarine, but again only in small quantities; and avoiding fatty cuts of meat and poultry. Also avoid palm and coconut oils. They are often found in blended vegetable oils so stick to the pure varieties.

  If you are normal weight for your height or under-weight, take care that by making these changes you do not lose weight.
- Tea and coffee consumption should be limited to a combined total of three cups or two mugs per day. Preferably abstain from these completely. Their caffeine content can aggravate symptoms of anxiety.
- If you suffer from fluid retention, then follow the advice about a low-salt diet, on page 243.
- Don't be afraid to eat more food in the week before your period. It is normal for appetite to increase and calorie intake to go up in the premenstrual week by as much as 20 per cent. Do this by allowing yourself more nutritious snacks rather than bingeing on sweets, chocolate, cakes, biscuits or bread.
- Limit your intake of bread. Some women with PMS seem

to improve dramatically if they completely cut out all wheat, oats, barley and rye from their diet. This is rather drastic, and many women find it easier to limit themselves to one or two slices of white bread per day, and one portion of white pasta per week.
- Do not consume wheat-containing or wheatbran-containing breakfast cereals. Rely upon rice- and corn-based cereals instead and increase their fibre content by adding fruit, nuts and seeds.

Premenstrual syndrome diet – sample menus

Here are some sample menus for you to make a start with:

Breakfast 1

rice crispies with chopped banana and crumbled pecan nuts
semi-skimmed milk
2 rice cakes with low-sugar jam
herb tea or dandelion coffee

Breakfast 2

2 boiled eggs or mushroom and tomato omelette
rice toast and low-sugar marmalade
fruit juice or herb tea

Breakfast 3

cornflakes with chopped pear and sunflower seeds
semi-skimmed milk
2 rice cakes and low-salt peanut butter
a glass of orange juice

Mid-morning snacks

fruit yoghurt
raw vegetables and humous or taramasalata
fruit and nuts

Lunch 1

jacket potato with tuna and sweetcorn
mixed salad

Lunch 2

tinned mackerel, tuna, sardine or cold meat (unsalted)
green salad
coleslaw

Lunch 3

vegetable omelette
watercress, fennel and lemon salad

Mid-afternoon snacks

rice cakes and low-sugar jam
rice toast with low-sugar peanut butter
nuts and raisins

Dinner 1

grilled or baked white fish
brown rice
fresh broccoli and sweetcorn
rhubarb and ginger mousse

Dinner 2

grilled lean chops
carrots
fresh greens
potatoes
baked bananas and low-fat yoghurt

Dinner 3

corn pasta with tuna and walnut cream sauce
mixed green salad
fresh fruit salad

Remember that premenstrual syndrome is best treated by dietary change in conjunction with the use of appropriate nutritional supplements and exercise. Counselling, certain drugs and hormonal treatments are also of value, and if your progress is not satisfactory then see your doctor for further advice and treatment.

Two useful books you might like to refer to are *Beat PMT Through Diet* and the *PMT Cookbook*, both by Maryon Stewart (published by Vermilion).

These books and other useful information are available from the Women's Nutritional Advisory Service. See page 339 for details.

CONCLUSION

By now hopefully, you will be able to determine the type of diet that is most suitable for you.

Remember that essentially you are going to be following the Very Nutritious Diet with perhaps one or more of the modifications. If you are in doubt about some of the modifications then stick with the basic diet to start with and after a few weeks, once you feel confident, make some of the other modifications depending upon your symptoms.

If, however, you have fatigue and other problems, such as eczema, nettle rash (urticaria), asthma, or migraine and irritable bowel syndrome then you may need to try the Exclusion Diet.

18

Exclusion diets

An exclusion diet may be an invaluable approach when chronic fatigue has persisted and no underlying physical cause has been found, or chronic fatigue is accompanied by several complaints that may be related to food allergy or intolerance such as migraine headaches, irritable bowel syndrome, asthma, nettle rash (urticaria) and eczema. Following a more formal Exclusion Diet, as opposed to the Very Nutritious Diet, may then be necessary.

Even if you haven't the classical or typical symptoms of allergy or intolerance, you may still benefit from an exclusion diet as there is now some evidence that intolerance to gluten may be associated with an increased risk of fatigue. Often, there may be a clue, such as the presence of minor bowel symptoms, including abdominal bloating with either diarrhoea or constipation. However, these symptoms may not have to be present for there still to be some mild degree of food intolerance contributing to your chronic fatigue symptoms.

WHO CAN DO THE DIET AND HOW
DO YOU DO IT?

It may be worth trying a partial exclusion diet provided that you fall into one of the two categories above, are not underweight, have no known associated serious illness, or do not need to follow a diet for some other reason, e.g. diabetes.

There are two types of exclusion diet to choose from. The Partial Exclusion Diet is not too restricted, and is relatively safe and easy to follow. The Full Exclusion Diet is more complicated and should be followed under the guidance of a doctor or dietician.

PARTIAL EXCLUSION DIET

The concept of a partial exclusion diet is to provide a nutritionally adequate diet that excludes the foods most commonly associated with intolerant or allergic reactions. These are detailed below, with the alternatives or substitutes that can be eaten in their place.

So, avoid the following beverages and foods:

Tea and coffee

These should be avoided completely, including the decaffeinated versions, if you have bowel symptoms. Use any of a variety of herbal teas or other low-tannin teas instead. Cut down on the tea and coffee gradually, otherwise withdrawal headaches and other symptoms may occur.

Alcoholic beverages

These should be avoided completely. Gin, vodka and white rum may be acceptable, as might the occasional glass of white wine. Consume them always with food and never on an empty stomach.

Wheat, oat, barley and rye

These cereals contain gluten. They should be avoided completely. This includes all bread, biscuits, cakes, pasta, pastry, pies, puddings, most breakfast cereals (except those containing rice and corn), semolina, cracked wheat, bulgar wheat, communion wafers, foods made with bread, bread-crumbs, wheat starch. Take care particularly with sausages, burgers, fish or other foods in batter, potato croquettes, chocolate bars containing a wafer, muesli bars, barley-based drinks or malted drinks, some soups, sauces, gravies and even some hot drinks from vending machines. Some sweets, e.g. liquorice or boiled sweets, may be rolled in fine wheat flour. Occasionally, some drugs, medicines or vitamin preparations may contain gluten as a filling agent.

This all sounds a bit drastic but there are now many acceptable alternatives to these grains.

Bread   Instead of ordinary bread you can eat rice cakes or gluten-free bread with spreads or make toast from rice bread. Rice cakes are now available in supermarkets and the bread can be ordered from your chemist or health food shop. Shop around as the prices do vary.

Pasta   Corn pasta is now available from health food shops. Also, some shops sell pasta and spaghetti made from brown rice.

Breakfast cereal Any rice or corn cereals will be fine, even the ordinary rice crispies and cornflakes from the super-market. (They do contain a little sugar but too little to worry about). Add some chopped fruit and some crumbled nuts to your cereal to make it a bit more wholesome.

Baking and cooking You will find that you can still make biscuits, cakes, pastry, sponge and pancakes using alter-native flours. It will take you a little time to experiment at first, to find the consistency that you like.

Brown rice flour is probably the best for making sponge. Make it up to the weight given in the recipe by mixing it with a little ground almond and a raising agent.

Savoury pancakes can be made with pure buckwheat flour. It is part of the rhubarb family, and tends to be quite heavy, so it can be mixed with a little white rice flour which is very light.

A crisp coating for fish or meat can be made with maize meal, which can be found in the health food shop. Coat the fish or meat with maize meal, then with beaten egg, and once again with maize meal. You can then bake, grill or even fry the food which when cooked should emerge with a crispy coat. You can also use gram (chick pea) flour, cornflour and many other alternatives that you will find in the health food shops.

Snacks It's nice to have something to crunch on when you are avoiding wheat. There are lots of corn products avail-able, but do remember to read the labels as some have added wheat. There are corn chips, crisps and wafers. Look in the Mexican section of the supermarket. Also, papadoms are fine, and little mini spiced papadoms are nice to nibble on or dip, but they do contain salt.

Milk products

This includes cow's milk and cheese, cream and yoghurt. Butter, which is composed mainly of fat, may be tolerated. The allergy or intolerance is often to the cow's milk protein and there may be an insignificant amount of this in butter, which is why it is more easily tolerated. Alternatively, if cow's milk products produce diarrhoea, the intolerance could be to lactose – milk sugar. This should therefore be avoided in all its forms. Note that many other foods contain cow's milk protein, including soups, sauces and many packaged foods. Again, look at the labels. If it mentions cow's milk or cheese, avoid them, but also avoid them if they say they contain skimmed milk, milk solids, non-fat milk solids, whey, caseinates, lactalbumin or lactose.

Many vegetarian margarines contain small amounts of cow's milk protein, so read the label. Unfortunately, many people who genuinely react to cow's milk, also react to sheep or goat's milk. It's therefore probably better to avoid these initially but they can be tried at a later date or at a time when you can hawkishly watch for any reactions.

The main alternative to cow's milk is soya milk. Calcium-enriched forms of soya milk are now available in many supermarkets and other food outlets. It is particularly important that growing children and women who are pregnant or breastfeeding use these calcium-enriched soya milk preparations. Additional calcium supplements may be necessary and you should consult your doctor about this if you need to avoid cow's milk products in the long term.

Salt

Salt in cooking, salt added to food and salty foods should be avoided if fluid retention is a significant problem, as detailed on page 244.

Foods containing additives

These should be avoided, but those most likely to cause adverse reactions include the azo-dye colouring agent, E102–155 (except E120, 140, 141, 150 and 153), E180, the benzoate preservatives E210–219, sulphites and sulphur dioxide E220–227, and monosodium glutamate, MSG, and its derivatives E621–623. Many preservatives and colouring agents are now naturally derived or are vitamins. Again, read the label carefully.

Benzoates and colouring agents can trigger nettle rash (urticaria), sulphites and colourings can aggravate asthma and colourings can also worsen or cause eczma especially in children.

Yeast-rich foods

The main foods rich in yeast include yeast extract preparations, e.g. Marmite, Vegemite, Barmene and other yeast extracts, stock cubes, vinegar, soy sauce and other fermented soy products, pickled foods, bread or other foods made with yeast extract, and alcoholic beverages. Some of these have already been excluded anyway. Dried fruits and over-ripe fruits may contain significant amounts of yeast and these are best avoided. Fruit juices that have spoiled, as may occur easily in warm weather if they are left out of the fridge, again can contain significant amounts of yeast and should be avoided. Yeast-free stock cubes are now available in some health food shops. Have fresh fruits and make sure that you drink only fresh fruit juices.

Fruit

Citrus fruits are fruits that come up most frequently in publications on food allergy and intolerance. However, adverse reactions to many other fruits have indeed been recorded. Often these are immediate reactions to fruits such as kiwi. Bananas and pears are reckoned to be particularly safe, but even adverse reactions to these are known. Tomatoes may need to be avoided. Those who react to raw tomatoes seem often to tolerate them cooked.

Nuts

Avoid peanuts (ground nuts), but other tree nuts, like almonds, walnuts, Brazil nuts, etc., can be eaten in moderation.

Vegetables

Severe adverse reactions to vegetables are rare. The most likely experience of an adverse effect is abdominal bloating and wind which may occur with some vegetables. It is difficult to make hard and fast rules about this, but some individuals may need to avoid peas, beans, lentils, red and green peppers, onions, garlic, leeks, cabbage, broccoli and cauliflower. This is particularly true if abdominal bloating and wind occur. Sometimes sweetcorn (maize) needs to be avoided too, but adverse reactions seem to occur relatively infrequently in UK residents, but more commonly in those living in North America, where the consumption of sweetcorn is much greater.

Egg and chicken

These do not need to be restricted unless you know that you react adversely to them. Eggs not infrequently produce eczema in children and here the reaction may be obvious. Cooked eggs, especially if included in a cake, for example, may be tolerated when plain egg is not.

Fish

Adverse reactions to fish, like eggs, can be severe and are often obvious. It may not be feasible to exclude fish or shellfish from this diet, unless you know or strongly suspect that you react adversely to them.

Meat

Again this does not have to be restricted unless you know or strongly suspect that it causes problems. Adverse reactions to meat and offal are not unknown and seem to be more likely with beef and pork.

Chocolate

In all its forms.

Foods that you know or suspect aggravate or cause your symptoms

Trust your own judgement. Remember that this diet is simply an educated guess, like all other exclusion diets. If you know or observe that a particular food causes problems for you, and has not already been listed, then avoid it. Even the best blood tests for food allergy may not pick up all types of allergic or intolerant reactions.

FOLLOWING AN EXCLUSION DIET

As already stated, the principle of the diet is that you follow it for a set time period. This should be for three to four weeks provided that the diet is not too difficult and you are not losing weight (unless this is desirable). If, after three to four weeks, there is no improvement then the diet should be abandoned and you should return to either your normal diet or the Very Nutritious Diet on pages 220–225. If, however, there is some good improvement in the level of physical or mental fatigue or in the associated symptoms then you should move on to the next stage where you reintroduce foods.

Reintroducing foods

The concept here is simple. Once your symptoms have improved follow this procedure:

- You choose a food group from the list below and add it back into your diet.
- Each food group is best added back at weekly intervals starting on a day when you do not have too many commitments for that day and the next two or three, in case there is an adverse reaction. The weekend or a Friday evening is often a good time to reintroduce foods especially if you are working.
- Eat a normal to large portion of the food or foods in question daily or nearly every day.
- If you feel unwell or notice any old symptoms returning during the reintroduction of a food or food group then stop eating that food and regard it as one to which you are allergic or intolerant until proven otherwise. It will need to be retested at a later date.
- Sometimes an adverse reaction might occur within an hour of eating a food whereas other times it may not affect you until the end of the week. Also it could take anything from a day to a week for any reaction to settle

down. Accordingly some parts of the diet will take longer than others to complete.

- If, when you add back a food, you experience only mild symptoms and are not sure if this is an adverse food reaction then continue with the food to the end of the week. By then it should be fairly clear to you whether it was an adverse reaction or not. If you are still not certain then either regard that food as one that upsets you and attempt to reintroduce it again at a later date, or have only very small amounts of the food once or twice per week.

- Be particularly careful when adding back wheat, other grains and dairy products. Reactions to these foods can be subtle and are often delayed for several days.

- Keep a written record of the foods you add back, any symptoms that are experienced, how long after first eating the food they occur and how long they take to resolve.

- If you have a bad reaction to a food don't be alarmed. It should settle down in a few days and it is perfectly acceptable to make use of painkilling drugs, steroid creams for eczema or medicines to settle the bowel if necessary. Do try and keep these to an effective minimum.

- If no adverse symptoms are experienced in the course of a week then you can fairly assume that that food is well tolerated and you can eat it normally adding it to your diet.

- Most people who react to one food also react to some others. Occasionally only one particular food or food group is found but this is more the exception rather than the rule. So if you do have a problem with one food don't think that you have found 'it'. Carry on and test out all the foods that you avoided in the first part of the diet.

What to do if you get into difficulties

You may get into difficulties. This happens occasionally and there are a number of possible reasons:

- You may have missed an adverse reaction to a food which you are now eating. Look over your diet from just before you were last doing well and see if you may have been eating something you shouldn't have by mistake.
- You may have had a flare up of your symptoms because of a genuine post-infective syndrome. This is unfortunate and is unavoidable.
- You may have developed some other problem such as a cold or flu. Again this is unavoidable and makes interpretation of the diet very difficult.
- You may have a mixed response with mild benefit because you have cut out foods that were genuinely upsetting you but with some deterioration because of a loss of nutritious foods or because of the strain of following the diet.

In these situations it is best to get some assistance from a doctor or dietician. If there was a point on the diet when you were doing particularly well then go back to it for a week or two and if that improves matters then continue adding foods, leaving off anything that you know or suspect upsets you.

Sometimes, but not that often, no adverse reactions are experienced! This can happen and it may well be that your body has simply got better or that some mild food sensitivities have faded into the background. Yes, sometimes people do get better automatically as the body has very substantial powers of recovery.

Foods to add back on the exclusion diet

This is a list of foods to be added back after three to four weeks on the first part of the exclusion diet. They should be added back at intervals of four days either in the order given or with a little modification to suit your personal preferences. Do not, however, alter the sequence given for 'wheat and other grains' as you may easily become confused. You don't have to add back everything. You can leave off those foods you never eat and those foods that you unquestionably know upset you, or that you know you don't like. When starting, many people like to try all the foods that they have missed the most. This often means tea and coffee, bread or chocolate. For this reason they are at the start of the list.

Tea or coffee

Don't have both, just one and only black or with soya milk or non-dairy whitener. You may want to try out milk first so that you can then try out a proper cup of tea or coffee.

Wheat and other grains

Follow this sequence carefully only going on to the next if the previous food was tolerated.

- White pasta without any egg. One portion on each of the four days. White flour can also be used for sauces and in cooking.
- Wholemeal pasta again without egg. One portion per day. Whole wheat breakfast cereal without any yeast is also allowed. Make sure that the pasta is made with wheat and does not contain dairy products or eggs.

Dairy products

Cow's milk, cream, yoghurt and butter.

Cheese

All types.

Citrus fruits

Fruits and their juices.

Meat

Beef or pork and their related offal if excluded.

Other meat

Pork or beef whichever had not been tried if relevant.

Coffee or tea

Whichever was not allowed before. Milk can be added if tolerated.

Alcoholic beverages

Only consume the ones that you were drinking before. Many traditional ales are very rich in yeast so if you react adversely to them take care with the next category.

Yeast-containing foods

Stock cubes, yeast extracts, e.g. Marmite, Bovril, Vegemite and Barmene. Savoury snacks and soups containing yeast provided the other ingredients are allowed or tolerated.

Oats

Oatmeal for porridge and oat flapjacks if the other ingredients are tolerated.

Peanuts (groundnuts)

Plain or salted if allowed. Not dry roasted which often contain many additives including monosodium glutamate.

Rye

This can be taken as pure rye bread – pumperknickel – and rye crispbreads.

Barley

This can be added to soups and stews. Many people who react to wheat may also react to oats, rye and barley as they all contain the protein gluten which seems to be a factor in such true allergic reactions. However, this is quite variable and it is often useful to test these grains individually.

Other fruits

Try reintroducing excluded fruits like tomato.

Vegetables

If any are excluded, these can be added back in groups, e.g. onion, leeks and garlic as one group; cabbage, broccoli and cauliflower as another; and beans as another.

Chocolate

Try plain if cow's milk is not tolerated.

Salt

If it has been excluded and has not already been tried.

Other foods

Any other foods that may have been excluded.

It is important to realise that it will take two and a half months to add back all of these foods if they are all relevant to you. This is only really worth doing if there has been substantial improvement in your symptoms in the first part of the diet.

Such diets are not to be undertaken lightly. It is often best to take time to prepare carefully for them, planning meals, menus and making shopping lists before you begin.

WHERE TO NEXT?

After you have tested all the foods and decided which ones you can't tolerate, you should continue to avoid the suspect list for the next few weeks or months. If this means not eating a large number of foods that were staples in your diet then care needs to be taken to ensure that your new diet is adequate and that you do not lose an excessive amount of weight.

If you go without milk and cheese for more than a few weeks you may well not be getting enough calcium and will therefore need to take a supplement of about 500 milligrams per day. This is particularly important for women around the age of fifty or older and for young people under the age of eighteen. It would also be relevant for any woman who became pregnant or was breastfeeding whilst on a restricted diet. Many doctors also recommend that anyone who follows an exclusion diet for a long time or lands up on a restricted diet in the long term should take a modest strength multivitamin and mineral supplement.

After a few months it is prudent to retest some of the foods that previously upset you, one by one as before. If they still do, you should continue to avoid them. However, very often small amounts of previously untolerated foods can be eaten, especially if only consumed a few times each month. It can be very useful to know that you can relax your diet every so often when going out, eating with friends or at home.

If you have found or suspect that you have many allergies or intolerances that are persistent then you should definitely discuss this with your doctor if you have not done so already. Specialist dietary advice can be invaluable and some types of allergic reactions can be partly or fully controlled using some very mild drugs.

FULL EXCLUSION DIET

This is included for interest and completeness. It is not intended that you should follow this kind of diet without expert guidance from your doctor or dietician. This type of diet is usually only followed for one to two weeks and then either foods are added back into the diet step-by-step or, if there has been no improvement in the first part of the diet, then the diet is abandoned completely.

Which foods are allowed?

Only the following foods are allowed and all other foods and beverages are prohibited.

- Meat: lamb, turkey and rabbit and their offal.
- Fish: choose two out of cod, plaice, salmon or trout.
- Vegetables: carrots, swedes, turnips, parsnips, spinach, lettuce, cucumber and courgettes.
- Fruit: pears without their skins, bananas, mangoes, pomegranates, papaya (pawpaw) and melons. Take care that the fruit is not over-ripe.
- Rice: white or brown and rice cakes.
- Vegetable oils: such as sunflower, safflower, corn, soybean, olive or rapeseed, and pure margarines made from them and not containing any dairy products.
- Water: tap if good quality, filtered tap or bottled if not.
- Herbal teas.
- Sugar: small amounts of sugar and honey are allowed.
- Salt: small amounts are allowed unless you have fluid retention.
- Soya milk: this is sometimes allowed and is essential for children.

This kind of diet is not nutritionally adequate and should not be followed for more than a week or two. It may be prudent for some people on this type of diet to take a multivitamin preparation. There are also great difficulties if you are a vegetarian or a vegan and need to follow such a restricted diet. You will certainly need expert guidance.

If you experience a significant improvement in your symptoms on this type of diet then you will need to add foods back in a controlled fashion as described in the Partial Exclusion Diet on pages 265–8.

19

Improving your mental outlook

In medicine, treatment can take a wide variety of forms. At one end of the treatment spectrum there is the so-called 'magic bullet' effect. Antibiotics, powerful drugs or even the correction of a severe vitamin or mineral deficiency can produce a magic bullet effect. Doctors and patients alike love to see this kind of therapy in action. It makes the junior doctors feel like gods and the patients bless the ground upon which they walk. Alas, this scenario is rare in medicine. At the other not so pleasant end of the spectrum the doctor says to the patient, 'It's all in your mind, you just have to pull your socks up.' Here the responsibility for recovery falls totally to the patient which many find a near impossible task when left to their own devices.

Occasionally, when treating chronic fatigue syndrome, there will be the case that responds to a magic bullet treatment. However, for the majority of patients there is good evidence now that the best way forward is to consider a number of treatments including psychological and lifestyle factors, and take a 'middle of the road view'. As has been mentioned many times in earlier parts of the book, lifestyle stresses and personal outlook may have a big influence on physical health and one's own powers of recovery.

GETTING BETTER IN MIND AND BODY

The first thing to acknowledge is that you *can* get better, indeed you are likely to get better. A number of studies from responsible researchers have demonstrated that there is a significant spontaneous recovery rate in chronic fatigue syndrome and that many other sufferers can be helped by self-help measures that address both physical and psychological aspects. Unfortunately some of the most chronic and severe cases receive the greatest media coverage. Whilst no one can promise that this won't happen to you, there seems little point dwelling on it and viewing yourself as a 'helpless victim'. Being pessimistic will simply stand in the way of any possible recovery.

Take a good exterior look at your life. Work out which aspects of life you find stressful. List them, then look at ways that you can adjust your lifestyle and avoid stressful situations. Consider the areas of your working career, family, friends, personal relationships, finances and social activities. The best way to start solving problems in these areas is to talk about them with either the people involved or a good friend. Often just talking through a situation can help you see the way out. If this is not enough as, for example, in the case of marital or financial difficulties you would be better off seeking professional advice.

Try not to be introverted. Chronic disability and pain often result in a reduced ability to see things from an exterior point of view. This introspection tends to increase the feelings of disability and apathy. Often, people with chronic fatigue have become less physically and mentally active than they previously were. If you are over the acute phase of your illness, begin now to think of ways in which you can build up your level of mental and perhaps physical activity gradually. Perhaps there are some hobbies that you stopped doing, books you wanted to read, friends you wanted to contact, letters you wanted to write, even places you wanted to visit. You might only be able to indulge in these activities for a short while at a time, perhaps ten or fifteen minutes in the morning and for the same time in the afternoon or evening. As with physical exercise, gradually increase the amount that you can cope with mentally. Try to involve yourself with others, perhaps playing some games with the children or young friends.

Make sure you have lots of variety in your day; boredom increases the level of introspection. Variety is truly the spice of life. Seek pleasure whenever you can. Hedonism – the pursuit of pleasure – is an underrated philosophy! This does not mean pleasure at the expense of others but with others. Think of all those things that have given you pleasure in the past and work out ways in which you could indulge in them now. A good meal, a chat with a friend, looking over some old photos or whatever brings you pleasure. It is easy to feel withdrawn and unhappy because of your ailment, but pleasure, laughter and even humour may prove to be stimulants to the immune system and certainly are tonics for one's spirit.

Try and build activities into a daily schedule. Having a regular daily schedule that includes time for getting up in the morning, time for meals, time for physical and mental activities and time for rest when necessary is important. The discipline of a routine is essential in hospitals and other caring institutions. It may be even useful to write out a timetable for yourself for the coming week. That way you won't have to be bored or frustrated thinking what to do next.

Be patient with yourself. Realise that progress may be slow and try and adjust your expectations accordingly. You may already have done this or perhaps you are slowly coming to terms with it. For many, chronic fatigue is an uncomfortable experience, particularly those who have led successful, go-ahead existences without more than the occasional day's illness. Your past reactions and responses that dealt with minor illnesses may be inappropriate when dealing with chronic fatigue. Education, personal realisation and adjustment are the first steps to making the changes which will allow you to respond in a positive way.

If you still have worries or problems express them. It is no use bottling them up. However, try to be as pleasant as possible to those around you. They too may have to share some of the burden of your fatigue. If you do want to discuss difficulties then try to balance this with pleasant or complimentary comments. Remember the adage 'do as you would be done by'.

If you still have concerns or worries about your physical health that you have not discussed with your doctor then do so. By now you should have an idea that there are many physical and psychological factors that can contribute to fatigue. Investigating, addressing and correcting them is an important part of many people's recovery plan and your own GP can refer you for psychological and social support as well as for further medical assessment.

Finally do not despair. The human body is extremely robust and it usually takes more than one nutritional deficiency and certainly more than one physical illness to really produce lasting ill-health. The human body is built to work even though some parts are malfunctioning. That is its beauty and its strength.

Hopefully the foregoing advice will help you to accept

what responsibilities you comfortably can in relation to your treatment plan. The support of your family doctor plus counsellors, psychologists, psychiatrists, etc., is invaluable in these situations.

20

The role of exercise

Physical exercise is a difficult subject to address. Traditionally, rest has, until recently, been a mainstay of treatment in chronic fatigue states. The condition 'neurasthenia' – weakness of the nervous system – was first described in the mid-nineteenth century and this term has been in common medical usage until recent times. The 'rest cure' for neurasthenia was popularised at the end of the last century with great success. Excessive rest, however, brings its own problems. Muscles waste, their ability to do work reduces and weight gain can occur. Thus lack of normal physical exercise can aggravate some of the loss of muscle function that occurs in chronic fatigue. This is unavoidable during an acute infection or when there is an exacerbation (acute worsening) of chronic symptoms or a new infection. Prolonged physical inactivity, however, has never been shown to benefit people with chronic fatigue. So unless there are significant underlying muscle or nerve problems it is unlikely to be of any help. Essentially rest should, like use of sedative drugs, be kept to a minimum. The difficulty comes in determining when it is best to begin increasing the level of physical activity.

It may be useful to break down the approach to exercise in chronic fatigue states into several stages:

- First ensure that there is no active infection or illness. Weight loss, fever or muscle wasting could all mean that physical exercise is quite inappropriate.
- Also exclude any hidden physical illness as given in Part 1 of the book (pages 53–86).
- It is probably prudent to make sure that your diet is adequate and that in particular there are no deficiencies of nutrients that are known to influence muscle function, especially vitamin B1 (thiamine) and other B complex vitamins, potassium and magnesium and to a lesser extent iron and possibly zinc. Following the Very Nutritious Diet approach (see pages 218–253) with supplements for an eight-week period should help correct the majority of any mild or moderate deficiencies.

At some stage you should be ready to begin exercising and to do this you should set a goal. This is not a long-term goal aimed at 'complete recovery' but a short-term goal. By the term 'exercising' I am referring really to any kind of physical activity. This includes simply walking out into the garden or round to a neighbour's house, even just to the car to be taken out for a drive. For those who are not so badly affected, longer walks or gentle sporting activities – especially swimming – could be considered. Many individuals, when first starting out, find that they have to rest for several days after some kind of physical activity, for example a five- or ten-minute walk may only be taken on alternate days or once in three days. However, by continuing regularly, even at these intervals, many people have found that they have been able to increase their level of physical activity gradually and feel all the better for it.

WHICH EXERCISE?

It is important to choose a type of physical activity that is easy for you to do, pleasant and feasible for you to carry out.

The benefits of exercise are over the long term. There is usually no benefit in the first few weeks other than that invaluable sense of achievement. It is vital, if not essential, that your success with exercise outweighs the difficulties. In the longer term, the majority of us only do things that bring us pleasure. Hedonism – the philosophy of enjoying pleasure – is not a dirty word provided that you are not doing it at someone else's expense. Think of what types of physical activity you have enjoyed in the past, and if they are feasible try them again. Perhaps there was a sporting activity that you were good at in your youth. Most middle-aged people will not take up new sporting activities but will simply return to those from their past that have been pleasurable.

GRADUALLY INCREASE YOUR LEVEL OF PHYSICAL ACTIVITY

Select a gentle but increasing target. For example, if you are able to go out for a walk for ten minutes on alternate days increase this by two to three minutes every fortnight. After twelve weeks you will be up to twenty minutes on alternate days. That is quite a socially useful distance as it would allow most people to either walk to the shops or once driven to the shops to go shopping, perhaps with rests in between. Acknowledge the fact that it may be as long as six months or a year before your physical activity level has returned to anything like normal.

CHOOSE ACTIVITIES THAT BRING YOU INTO CONTACT WITH OTHER PEOPLE

Going for a walk with a friend, going with your children, grandchildren, partner or relatives will all help to increase the level of pleasure and encourage you to continue.

ESTABLISH A LONGER-TERM GOAL

Once you have had some success with your short-term goals building up your level of physical activity and perhaps trying a variety of different types of exercise, consider what your long-term goal should be. If you have never been very sporty as a young person then it is unlikely that you will achieve full body fitness. This would require, for example, forty minutes' strenuous aerobic exercise three times a week. Of those who have been physically active and who have then developed an infection or illness in chronic fatigue syndrome, many will want to return to their previous level of health and fitness and will consider that they are 'ill' until they have done so. I have seen several patients like this. If, however, you have had 'couch potato' tendencies for most of your life, acknowledge now that this is not the best way to continue. Even maintaining a modest level of exercise, for example a thirty to forty minute daily walk, will improve physical fitness. Don't forget that physical exercise has benefit not only for your heart and circulation but also helps depression, improves sleep and helps weight loss when combined with an appropriate calorie-restricted diet.

When you feel up to it try a gentle workout for a few minutes a few times per week and gradually build yourself up physically. The YMCA have produced a twelve-minute video called 'Y Plan'. It is certainly worth having a go at this when you feel ready.

WHEN TO BEGIN

There is a time when it is appropriate and a time when it is inappropriate to start exercising. Judging the changeover may be difficult and guidance is often necessary, although a degree of trial and error is also required. If you have been physically fit in the past, and you have none of the conditions that will prevent you from beginning to exercise (see page 278), then bite the bullet and begin gradually. In this way the liabilities are kept to a minimum. Once you have begun to reap the benefits of exercise you will feel more confident.

There is now good medical evidence that patients with chronic lung and heart disease who were previously advised to 'take it easy' are better off if they take a modest amount of physical exercise on a regular, preferably daily basis. This is a complete change in medical advice, but then we should be getting used to that! Sometimes we just have to get it wrong before we get it right!

MENTAL EXERCISE

Just as one needs physical exercise to maintain physical health we also need to maintain mental activity in order to retain our mental abilities. Loss of concentration and reduction in memory are common complaints with chronic fatigue syndrome. Maintaining some kind of mental activity such as reading, listening to the radio, doing a crossword, playing games like chess, draughts or word games may all be helpful ways of stimulating and maintaining mental activity. Often these activities can only be undertaken for brief periods – a few minutes or half an hour. Just as eating a good diet, getting fresh air and some exercise is part of your convalescence programme, so is using your mind. Although as far as we know it does not have any direct effects on physical health, by maintaining your morale it can help reduce the tendency of slipping into a 'diseased frame of mind'. Unfortunately the ubiquitous television and video have dominated many people's leisure time. Prolonged viewing of television is now associated with reduced reading and educational ability in children so beware of its mind-numbing effects.

Make a list of your interests and hobbies and work out how you can pursue some of them even if only to a limited degree. In this way your mental activities will be maintained. Try and involve others – friends, partner, children or other relatives – so that this helps to maintain social contact.

If you are well on the road to recovery but are not employed think about adult education classes during the day-time or evening. By now you should have got the message, 'Don't stew in your own juice'. It is unlikely to do you any good.

21

Pills and potions – what to take and when

NUTRITIONAL SUPPLEMENTS

Many of you reading this book may have already tried taking a variety of nutritional supplements and perhaps some have experienced a degree of benefit. It is best to consider these rationally rather than to just take a hotch-potch of vitamins and minerals as quite a number are of proven benefit in chronic fatigue where a deficiency exists.

Multivitamins

These come in a variety of strengths, usually providing at least the recommended daily allowance (RDA) of essential vitamins together with some minerals. They certainly should be taken by anyone with significant weight loss; ill elderly people (over the age of sixty-five); those on a restricted diet;

and those with a continued fever of unknown cause. There
are a wide variety to choose from and you may need to take
advice from your doctor, pharmacist or nutritional supplement supplier. As a general rule the dosage of the vitamin B
complex vitamins should be at least at the level of the
Recommended Daily Allowance (RDA) or Referenced
Nutrient Intake (RNI). Those studies that have shown
benefits of multivitamin supplements have usually been
conducted over at least three months so don't expect too
instant results.

High-dose vitamin B complex

High doses of vitamin B complex may be worth considering
if you fit one or more of the following categories:

- You have a high alcohol consumption (six or more units
  per day for men; four or more units per day for
  women).
- You have a history of or actual depression, anxiety or
  other mental symptoms.
- You have marked muscle weakness or pain on exercise.

The dosage of vitamins B1 (thiamine), B2 (riboflavin) and
vitamin B6 (pyridoxine) should normally be at a level of
between five and fifty times the Recommended Daily Allowance (RDA) or Referenced Nutrient Intake (RNI) levels.
Dosages can usually be reduced after two or three months
depending upon response, but high levels will need to be
maintained if alcohol consumption continues to be high.

Vitamin C – ascorbic acid

This will be contained in many multivitamin preparations.
  People at risk of deficiency are the elderly, especially

smokers or those eating a poor diet with little fruit and vegetables. A reasonable therapeutic dose is 500 milligrams daily for two months with reduced dosages thereafter. Taking up to three grams per day at the time of colds or other similar infections may be of modest benefit but the evidence for this is finely balanced. Though I have not personally found it to be of benefit I have met many patients who swear by it.

Magnesium

Some doctors would support the idea of giving supplements of magnesium to all of those with chronic fatigue syndrome. This would be a reasonable policy if future studies confirm that it routinely produces benefit. Fortunately it is an extremely safe supplement and the only people who should definitely not take it are those with kidney problems or chronic diarrhoea. It should be tried if you have:

• Chronic fatigue and a low level of red cell magnesium.
• Fatigue and PMS.
• Constipation.

If for any reason a red cell magnesium test can not be performed it is reasonable to try magnesium supplementation for a three- to four-month period.

There are many magnesium preparations available, including magnesium oxide, citrate, gluconate and amino acid. An effective dose is probably in the region of 200–400 mgs per day. Higher doses might give slightly loose stools or diarrhoea in some people and in this case should be reduced. Milk of magnesia is not a very well absorbed magnesium preparation and it's much less palatable than swallowing tablets.

For women with premenstrual syndrome Optivite, a

specialised multivitamin containing magnesium, is available and is perhaps worth considering (see pages 159–160).

Magnesium can also be given by injection as magnesium sulphate, 50 per cent solution, 2 millilitres intramuscularly (i.e. into the muscles). A reasonable dosage would be once or twice per week for eight weeks, but the injections can be a little painful. They are probably best reserved for those unable to tolerate oral supplements, which should be rare. Remember, magnesium balance may be influenced not only by taking magnesium but also by ensuring you have a good intake of protein in your diet and by limiting your intake of refined carbohydrates and possibly by the balance of other nutrients (see chapter Fatigue and Magnesium page 110).

Improvements in red cell magnesium levels have also been observed by giving high dose vitamin B6 which is best taken in the form of a vitamin B complex.

Iron

Ideally, if you have chronic fatigue syndrome you should have had your iron levels checked. Supplements of iron should be given to everyone with chronic fatigue syndrome who is iron deficient. A reasonable dosage is between 20–120 milligrams of iron element per day. Iron comes in many forms and the most popular are: ferrous sulphate, fumarate, gluconate. Many other iron preparations are available both in chemists and health food shops. There are tablet and liquid forms. The absorption of iron is enhanced by taking it with vitamin C (ascorbic acid) and the easiest way is to take the iron preparation with a glass of fruit juice, a piece of fruit or with vitamin C or multivitamins if you are also taking these. Its absorption is greatly reduced if it is taken with tea because of the tannin content.

A commonly prescribed preparation is ferrous sulphate –

200 milligram tablets and one tablet taken once or twice per day with fruit juice or fruit is a reasonable dosage providing 60 to 120 milligrams of iron.

Who should take iron supplements?

If you have iron deficiency; heavy or prolonged periods; if you are a female vegetarian; if you are ill and elderly; or if you are a young child you are advised to take multivitamins with iron, particularly if you fall within the last two categories.

If it is appropriate, you should continue to take iron for at least three months and possibly as long as six months depending on your circumstances. If you have continuing iron losses because of heavy periods it may be appropriate for you to continue to take regular modest doses of iron.

Iron should really be taken only by those people who are deficient. A very small percentage of the population accumulates excess quantities of iron during the course of a lifetime because of a condition called haemochromatosis which can run in families. For them it is particularly inadvisable to take iron tablets needlessly. Finally, even half a dozen adult iron tablets can cause serious ill effects if consumed by children, and all iron-containing preparations should be supplied in child-proof containers and kept out of their reach. In adults, iron may occasionally cause mild stomach side-effects. This is normally helped by reducing the dosage, taking it after meals and with fruit or fruit juice. Darkish discolouration of the stools is a normal occurrence in those taking large doses of iron.

Zinc

Zinc is perhaps the most important of the trace elements after iron. A few individuals with chronic fatigue and reduced resistance to infection may be deficient in zinc. This can be determined from a blood test to measure the level of zinc in the blood.

Who should take zinc supplements?

You are most likely to benefit from zinc supplements if you have evidence of a zinc deficiency e.g. low blood levels of zinc; if you have an acute sore throat (take zinc lozenges: one, three times per day); if you have poor resistance to infection; weight loss; or if you are ill and elderly.

Many forms of zinc are available: zinc sulphate, gluconate, citrate and amino acid chelate. A normal dosage is between 20 to 50 mgs of zinc daily. Higher doses may actually suppress the function of the immune system. Zinc is best absorbed if taken on an empty stomach. It should not usually be taken at the same time as iron which may interfere with its absorption. Occasionally zinc preparations cause minor stomach irritation and in this case it should be taken after eating fruit or a small snack.

It is usual to give supplements for three months, though longer administration of zinc and sometimes other trace nutrients may be necessary if the diet is restricted for any particular reason.

Evening primrose oil

Oil derived from the seed of the evening primrose plant is a rich source of certain essential fatty acids. The omega-6 series essential fatty acids are involved in cell structure and immune function. Deficiency in one of this series, gamma linolenic acid, has been found in some people with chronic fatigue syndrome and they often seem to respond well to evening primrose oil which is rich in this particular essential fatty acid.

Who should take evening primrose oil?

Those with chronic fatigue following an infection, who have not responded to other treatments and women with pre-menstrual breast tenderness are most likely to benefit.

Evening primrose oil (EPO) usually comes as 500 milli-grams or 1 gram capsules and dosage is 3 to 4 grams daily. It has been used successfully together with fish oils in a trial of patients with CFS. Dr Behan from Glasgow found 84 per cent of patients taking Efamol Marine for six months improved whilst only 22 per cent receiving placebo improved. It is usually given for three to four months and is best taken on a regular daily basis with food. There are virtually no side-effects but it is not advised that people with epilepsy take it as there are a few case reports that it can aggravate pre-existing epilepsy.

There are a variety of other preparations including borage seed oil (also known as starflower oil) and blackcurrant seed oil which have a similar composition to evening primrose oil. These have not, to my knowledge, been tried in chronic fatigue syndrome.

In the United Kingdom EPO can be prescribed on the National Health Service for benign breast problems but at the time of writing this book (1993) not for chronic fatigue syndrome itself.

Coenzyme Q10

This compound, which is not a vitamin but is related to vitamin metabolism, has been used successfully in certain fatigue states. The dosage used in one successful experiment was 60 milligrams of Coenzyme Q10 daily taken for four to eight weeks. It is, however, an expensive supplement. A significant amount can also be provided by eating a healthy well-balanced diet with plenty of vegetables.

DRUG THERAPY

This is a convenient point to consider some of the drugs that are used in the treatment of chronic fatigue syndrome. They can be broken down into various categories.

Antidepressants

There are several different types of antidepressants. One of the longest established are a group called tricyclic anti-depressants. They and other types may be useful for:

- Proven depression.
- Helping sleep – small doses given at night.
- Helping painful muscles – fibrositis or fibromyalgia – small doses have pain-relieving properties.
- Occasionally they may help prevent migraine headache.

There is some evidence to suggest that their effect on depression can be improved by combining them with modest doses of B complex vitamins. There are, however, no studies of their usage in chronic fatigue syndrome, and there are side-effects to contend with including: dry mouth, blurred vision, constipation and difficulty passing water.

High dosages should be avoided particularly if you are getting on in years and suffer with heart disease.

Tranquillisers and sleeping tablets

These have developed a rather bad reputation and not before time. Their excessive use by many doctors is a black chapter in the history of medicine. There are no studies that demonstrate their effectiveness in chronic fatigue states. Their use should really be confined to short-term treatment of severe anxiety and insomnia. Short-term use of low-dose benzodiazepines helps minimise the risk of developing dependency or experiencing adverse effects. There is considerable variation in the susceptibility of individuals in their sensitivity to these drugs.

Antibiotics

These are very useful agents in treating infections, especially bacterial and fungal ones. Certainly anyone with chronic fatigue syndrome who has a chronic hidden infection, e.g. sinus, dental, urinary or gynaecological infections, should be treated with an appropriate course of antibiotics.

If new infections arise during the course of the existing fatigue illness, they too should be treated with antibiotics when appropriate. Minor sore throats and ear infections may not always require antibiotic treatment but continuing fever, coughs and phlegm or a severe sore throat may often justify treatment. A full course should be taken for the appropriate length of time and occasionally a second course may be needed.

Fungal infections may also require treatment. Vaginal candida and other infections with candida have been associated with chronic fatigue states by some researchers. They respond to a number of anti-fungal agents, all of which are quite effective, but none is always so. They include nystatin (Nystan), clotrimazole (Canesten), econazole, miconazole, isoconazole, ketoconazole, itroconazole and fluconazol. They come in pessaries, cream and in tablet form. Ketoconazole, itroconazole and fluconazol when given by mouth are absorbed into the bloodstream and penetrate the vaginal and other tissues. They may be particularly useful when the vaginal thrush is resistant to more simple treatments. Occasionally prolonged courses may need to be given. In those who have recurrent or particularly difficult vaginal thrush other measures may be helpful (see page 175–186).

Antiviral drugs

Unfortunately there are very few drugs that are effective against viruses. There are a few preparations which are active against genital herpes such as inosine pranobex (Immunovir) and acyclovir (Zovriax). At present there is no proven effective antiviral treatment of value for patients with chronic fatigue syndrome. A trial of acyclovir showed no benefit when compared with placebo.

Immune stimulants and immune preparations

A number of drugs and natural compounds exist that can function as immune stimulants. At present they have no real part to play in people which chronic fatigue syndrome, though there has been the occasional case report of improvement when such compounds have been used in patients with evidence of chronic active viral infection. Treatment with gammaglobulins, which are blood proteins containing a wide variety of antibodies against different organisms, has also been used in two trials. An Australian trial reported a small degree of benefit but researchers in the UK in a similar but not identical trial did not find this to be the case.

At present most authorities do not consider that gamma-globulin is a useful treatment although it is used for the rare patients who have an actual lack of antibody proteins in their blood and evidence of repeated or chronic infections. It should not be forgotten that a variety of nutritional supplements including B vitamins, zinc and vitamin E have all been shown to result in improvements in immune function – usually in elderly subjects.

Immunisation

Though not exactly used in the treatment of chronic fatigue syndrome, this is an appropriate time to consider immunisation. The use of vaccines to immunise children has been one of the major breakthroughs in health in both developed and developing countries this century. Normal childhood immunisation should be given to those children unfortunate to have chronic fatigue syndrome, though some revision may be necessary in those with true immune deficiency syndromes. The elderly and those with heart disease and chest disease are now routinely immunised annually against influenza and the presence of chronic fatigue syndrome should not make any difference to this. Eventually vaccines against some of the viruses implicated in chronic fatigue syndrome may be developed which will hopefully become a useful way of reducing the percentage of people who are affected.

22

What complementary medicine has to offer

There is a limit to what we know as 'orthodox' medicine can offer the person who has been suffering with chronic fatigue, with no apparent underlying cause. Whilst those of us with a strong constitution can probably expect to recover naturally in time, sitting waiting to feel better is not a desirable pastime. There are a number of very valuable complimentary therapies that have a considerable amount to offer the chronic fatigue sufferer. Many of these therapies are based on sound ancient principles and have been used for generations. Unlike conventional medicine which tends to address conditions, the complementary therapies concentrate more on treating symptoms and aim to stimulate the body's own natural healing process.

When you are feeling tired and frustrated, the thought of exploring the world of holistic medicine can be a daunting prospect. There are so many different kinds of therapies and equally many different kinds of therapists. To make life easy for you I have chosen a number of disciplines that I feel would be worth investigating further.

ACUPUNCTURE

Acupuncture is a 5,000-year-old Chinese healing system which is still widely practised in China today. It uses pressure points on the body that are related to particular organs or functions to stimulate the energy flow through channels which are called 'meridians'. Chinese medicine determines a person's health or lack of it directly in terms of their vitality or lifeforce, and this vital force is called Qi (pronounced chi). This word encompasses both the general sense of energy, liveliness, health, vitality, resistance to disease, and a much more specific sense of the strength and efficiency of organic function within the body.

According to the Chinese, the Qi of each organ can be assessed by diagnostic means. Each organ has its own Qi. According to Chinese medical theory the lung Qi encompasses both breath and the breathing ability of the lungs and their power to transfer the breath and other sources of energy into the body. The lungs help to circulate Qi around the body and also have the power to transform the air and sources of air into vital substances.

Chinese medicine regards blood as the material foundation of all the different body tissues. All body tissues draw from the blood, and tissues draw energy from the Qi.

Acupuncture would regard symptoms of fatigue as a deficiency syndrome. The practitioner would be looking for deficiency of Qi or the lifeforce in the blood.

Diagnostic approach

When you go to see an acupuncturist you can expect a full history of your condition to be taken. They will assess your constitutional strength and try to understand the factors which have contributed to your illness. This may include details about hereditary and childhood predisposing factors, past health problems or more recent illnesses and particularly any illnesses or other life changes associated with the tiredness. Examples of these changes could be:

- Pregnancy or childbirth.
- Change of job.
- Redundancy.
- Menopause.
- Viral infections.
- Accidents.
- Shock.

The implication is that not only can physical illnesses deplete the vital source but also the stresses and strains of life itself.

Examination

During the examination the practitioner will be taking your pulse in different parts of the body, examining your tongue, looking at your complexion, listening to your voice and will ask you questions about your diet, sleep and your bowel habits.

If your Qi is deficient it is likely that you will find it difficult to keep warm, feel too tired to get things done, feel breathless, find it difficult to climb stairs, perhaps be tired in the morning and generally suffer from a lack of energy. The acupuncturist will select points on your body which by stimulating will help to increase the level of Qi and improve your energy levels.

A qualified acupuncturist will be concerned that you follow a good diet and that you take regular exercise and adequate rest as appropriate, as all these factors play an important part in your recovery.

Properly qualified acupuncturists take care to use sterilised needles to prevent the risk of transferring hepatitis and HIV (the AIDS virus).

If you don't happen to know of a good acupuncturist you can find the name of a registered practitioner by contacting the British Acupuncture Register and Directory or the Council for Acupuncture. Both of these addresses are listed on page 340. Medical studies now indicate that acupuncture can be an effective treatment for pain relief.

Shiatsu massage or acupressure

Shiatsu is a Japanese word meaning finger pressure. It is the name given to one of the oldest forms of healing – healing with the hands. It is very simple. It uses a few techniques, a sustained gentle pressure on various points on the body with the thumb, hand or arm, or a simple rotation or movement of the limbs. These movements are intended to encourage the energy to flow through the channels in the body in a similar way to acupuncture.

If you can't face the thought of the acupuncturist's needles then Shiatsu might be a confrontable alternative for you to explore. Shiatsu is now widely practised in this country and to find a registered practitioner you can contact the Shiatsu Society which is listed in the useful address section on page 340.

Suggested reading

An excellent book on Shiatsu with lots of demonstration pictures is, *The Book of Shiatsu – Vitality and Health Through the Art of Touch* by Paul Lundberg (published by Gaia). You could also try *Shiatsu* by Ray Ridolfi, published by Optima.

HOMOEOPATHY

Homoeopathy is one of the most established types of complementary medicine and is particularly well established in the United Kingdom and has long been a favourite of the Royal Family. Dr Samuel Hahnemann, a German physician in the late eighteenth and early nineteenth centuries, was the first to describe in detail the system and practice of homoeopathy. From his own observations, he considered that diseases best responded to particular treatments on the basis of like treating like. In other words, diseases tend to respond to treatments that can cause symptoms, that are in some way similar to the condition that one is treating. Homoeopathy literally means 'like the disease'. This was a system, therefore, for selecting medicines that might be effective for a particular type of illness.

In Dr Hahnemann's day, many of the drugs and compounds available were quite poisonous, and so he went on to formulate very dilute forms of quite potent compounds. Thus a homoeopathic practitioner would select a very dilute form of medicine, which when given in its concentrated form, might produce symptoms of the disease that he or she is trying to treat. Curiously, there are some examples of this in conventional medicine. Immunisation, for example, involves giving a weakened or dilute form of the virus or germ so that the immune system of the body is stimulated to resist any future contact with that infecting organism. Homoeopathy over the years has gained a reputation, therefore, for being a gentle and natural way of stimulating the body's own powers of recovery.

Is homoeopathy effective?

Though homoeopathic remedies have long been popular with the general public and even the Royal Family in the United Kingdom, doctors and scientists have been sceptical about its use. Only in recent years have proper scientific studies been conducted to test the effectiveness of homoeopathy. Some, but not all, have demonstrated the reasonable effectiveness of homoeopathic preparations when compared with dummy or placebo tablets. A review of these trials in the *British Medical Journal* in 1991 by a group of Dutch researchers concluded that on the whole modest support could be given to the use of homoeopathic preparations in certain conditions.

Homoeopathic remedies are particularly favoured for young children when conventional drugs cannot be tolerated and no other effective treatment has been found. They are also useful for patients who have many symptoms, but little in the way of a clearly treatable disease or for those unable to tolerate or who are unresponsive to drug therapy. This is often the case in patients with chronic fatigue. Modern medicine does not always have an answer for the symptoms that sometimes accompany chronic fatigue, and temporary and possibly long-term relief may be obtained by trying different homoeopathic preparations.

Doctors and other practitioners who use homoeopathy often take a very detailed history from the patient about their illness, symptoms, aggravating and relieving factors, diet and lifestyle. The system of medicine as proposed by Dr Hahnemann was in fact quite holistic and did not just rely upon the use of homoeopathic remedies. It may be useful to quote him from his writings of nearly 200 years ago, 'If a patient complains of one or more trivial symptoms that have been only observed a short time previously, the physician should not regard this as a fully developed disease that requires serious medical aid. A slight alteration in the diet and regimen [daily routine], will usually suffice to dispel such an indisposition.' Many cases of mild chronic fatigue would fall into this category. Here was a doctor who was clearly in tune with his patients, and had a deep understanding of illness.

Homoeopathic preparations for fatigue

Homoeopathic preparations come either in the form of tablets, granules, powder and occasionally as liquids. Usually small tablets of milk sugar (lactose) are impregnated with a liquid containing a very dilute and energised form of the original medicine. The dilution is denoted by number 6, 12, or 30, and the suffix 'C' or 'X' further indicates the strength. Curiously, unlike conventional medicine, the strength of the medicine is less important than choosing the right remedy.

Remedies for acute illness

Here are a dozen or so homoeopathic remedies that may be useful, either in acute infections, or chronic fatigue.

Ferr. Phos. (ferrum phosphoricum) A remedy for the early stages of a cold, with a stuffy or runny nose, dizziness, pale complexion, fever and general sensitivity. Typically, it is useful for symptoms that are worse at night or on exposure to the cold.

Gelsemium (gelsemium sempervirens) A remedy for flu and colds. Sneezing, sore throat, muscular aches and pains, headaches, lack of thirst – even with a fever – is part of the picture for this remedy. It is particularly suited to nervous, excitable individuals who have difficulty coping with life stresses.

Merc. Sol. (mercurius solubilis) Sore throat and cold remedy, especially if the mouth is full of saliva. Mouth ulcers or a sore mouth are also features.

Bryonia (bryonia alba) A remedy for a dry, painful, especially chesty cough. There is a thirst for cold drinks.

Remedies for chronic illness

I will broadly divide these into remedies where muscular aches and pains are common, remedies for depression, and remedies for chronic fatigue.

Remedies for aches and pains

Apis. Mel. (apis melifica) Literally, a useful remedy for rheumatism, aches and pains and swelling, including fluid retention. Listlessness and fatigue may also be symptoms.

Rhus. Tox. (rhus toxicodendron) A remedy derived from poison ivy. Classically one for painful, swollen and stiff joints, where the pain worsens on initial movement, but improves gradually thereafter. Symptoms tend to improve during warm weather.

Depression

Lycopodium (lycopodium clavatum) Fatigue, dislike of exercise, cravings, especially for sweet foods, fear of failure and wanting to be alone are symptoms that would suggest this remedy.

Nat. Mur. (natrum muriaticum) A remedy for the pale and weak. In historical times, this was a remedy for 'chlorosis' – anaemia – see pages 92–109. Chronic fatigue with moodiness, irritability, dislike of sympathy, headache, weak and stiff but not painful muscles are symptoms that would suggest this remedy. Also it can be used for colds, with a profuse runny nose.

Pulsatilla A remedy for the pale, frail female with changeable symptoms. Good for those who do not tolerate stress well. Also a useful remedy for thick catarrh from the nose or throat. Aversion to fat or greasy foods is said to be typical of those for whom this remedy is suited.

Swollen painful glands

Kali. Iod. A remedy for painful, swollen glands, fatigue and an acute cold.

Phytolacca Another remedy for swollen, inflamed glands. Useful also for tonsillitis and sore throats, rheumatic pains, fever and chills. This is a remedy that matches the picture of glandular fever and many virus infections.

This is just a selection of some of the 2,000 homoeopathic remedies that are available. Though homoeopathic remedies can be self-prescribed, there is no substitute for seeing a homoeopathic physician. Homoeopathic remedies can be prescribed for a short-lived illness such as a cough or cold, or in those with chronic fatigue who have been thoroughly assessed already by their doctor and/or specialist.

Homoeopathic remedies can be prescribed on the National Health Service. There are several NHS homoeopathic hospitals and clinics in the United Kingdom.

Suggested reading

'Homoeopathy for the Family' is a booklet produced by the Homoeopathic Development Foundation, Ltd. It is obtainable from HDF and many pharmacies.

HERBAL MEDICINE

According to the WHO (World Health Organisation), in the world as a whole approximately 85 per cent of people have access to so called 'primate' whole plan medication. 'Orthodox' drug-based medicine would thus be seen as fringe in many areas. People have been taking herbs as long as we have been eating – it is a subject as old as nutrition itself. Our ancestors, the hunter-gatherers, used to experiment with berries and fruit as remedies to their ailments on a trial and error basis. It was the womenfolk who usually discovered the remedies as men were not involved in tending the land until the advent of the heavy plough.

Plants fall into three distinct categories:

- *Drug-like* Some have effects on tissues that like drugs are predictable and substantial.
- *Alternative* These don't have drug-like activity and yet they have healing properties possibly because of stimulatory effects.
- *A combination* These fall between the two. An example is camomile which should belong in the second category, but it alters tissue state.

There are plenty of plants that have stimulating properties without being addictive, and there are hundreds of different strategies, and so finding the correct plant to suit each individual is an art learned over many years of study.

Herbs can also help to strengthen the immune system and fight infection. The most important group of herbs are those with antiviral properties. Plants themselves contain a variety of compounds that help the plant resist attack by viruses and fungi. These compounds are found together with minerals, vitamins and enzymes in many plants. A common example of a plant with antiviral properties is garlic. These immune-stimulating herbs can help to improve the body's ability to fight infection.

Herbs and fatigue

When you go along to see a medical herbalist you can expect to be asked lots of questions about your medical history including questions about depression, anaemia, allergies and other diseases. As well as helping to overcome your symptoms the herbalist will be looking at improving your immune system and cell function at a tissue level.

As there are so many different remedies it is not just a simple matter of saying take X, Y and Z to help you over your symptoms. The herbalist would need to consider your individual situation. However, there are certain herbs that he or she may be considering to help overcome fatigue, for example:

- St John's wort
- Vervain
- Yarrow
- Echinacea
- Stinging nettle

- Ginger
- Calendula
- Gypsywort
- Damiana
- Sage
- Valerian
- Prickly ash bark

There are also plants which might make matters worse so it is really important to seek professional advice. You can obtain a list of medical herbalists by contacting the National Institute of Medical Herbalists and you will find the address on page 340.

OSTEOPATHY AND CRANIAL OSTEOPATHY

Osteopaths believe that our structure governs our function to a large extent. If bones and muscles are tense or strained and if posture is poor, then it can have a direct effect on our general well-being.

Looking at the body as a whole – particularly at the back and the head – if there are restrictions where soft tissue is tight or bones misaligned there may be a reduction in the blood flow to tissues, which osteopaths believe can in turn cause congestion as the return flow is also restricted. Toxins are thought to accumulate producing symptoms of tiredness, headaches and other problems that relate to the central nervous system. That is the theory.

When you visit an osteopath once again you can expect to talk about any illnesses or accidents you have had from the time of your birth. You can also expect a physical examination to see how your joints move, how your muscles balance, how you walk and to check your general posture.

Cranial osteopaths in particular believe that women sometimes have a fixed pelvis after childbirth which can have an effect on their hormones.

Also, they consider that the membranes around the brain and spinal cord can become 'tight' and cause ill-health. Relaxation, massage and movement are the recommended ways of helping. Only qualified osteopaths can train to become cranial osteopaths. They provide very gentle treatment which helps the body back to normal function.

To find your nearest osteopath you can contact the British School of Osteopathy or the Cranial Osteopathic Association, details of these organisations are on page 340.

You will find that qualified practitioners of all these disciplines are often very knowledgeable and caring. They are trained to recognise when conventional medicine would perhaps be more appropriate and are usually very happy to work alongside your own doctor.

It is difficult to make firm recommendations about any of them as no studies of these complementary methods have been undertaken in fatigue. However, many people with a wide range of health problems have reported benefit, so they are all worth considering. As with conventional medicines and nutritional approaches let yourself be the judge. After all, if it works for you then that is the best test.

I hope that with the information I have given you and the help you receive from your doctor, you will be able to work your way back to optimum health in time. Be patient, Rome wasn't built in a day! You will be all the more grateful for your health when it is restored.

APPENDIX

Assessment of patients with chronic fatigue

It may be useful to outline some of the tests and assessments available for people with chronic fatigue and those, in my opinion, that should virtually be performed as routine. This advice is based upon the findings of many well-conducted studies, details of which appear at the end of this chapter, as well as my own experience.

With these tests in mind, I am referring always to people whose level of fatigue has been prolonged – for at least three months – and has been severe enough to disrupt their work or domestic lifestyle. If there has been an acute illness such as glandular fever or a severe bout of gastro-enteritis that triggered the fatigue, a detailed investigation is rarely required. These tests are more useful when people experience a gradual onset of severe fatigue which followed a trivial illness or appeared out of the blue.

Assessment is based on history, examination and laboratory investigations. We have already considered the history in much detail. The questions asked in the questionnaires from previous chapters cover many of the most important aspects of your history apart from your own perception of the problem.

EXAMINATION

A thorough medical examination is a cornerstone of good practice. It will include an examination of the heart, circulation, chest, abdomen, back, limbs, mouth, throat, nose, ears, eyes, skin including hair, nails, lymph glands and the nervous system. It is not done in five minutes but can be done in ten to fifteen minutes. More detailed assessments of muscle function and neurological examination can take a further fifteen minutes and are only usually necessary if the symptoms or initial examination warrant it.

An attempt should be made by the examining doctor to look for signs of nutritional deficiency including changes in skin quality, flattened, upturned or brittle finger nails, cracking at the corners of the mouth, smoothness or redness of the tongue, red greasy skin at the sides of the nose or outer angles of the eyes and other less common features. Most of these physical signs are caused by lack of vitamin B or iron, although there are other or additional causes for most of them.

Taking the temperature

If any fever is suspected it may be useful for you to take your own temperature. This is particularly important if there are symptoms of chills or if a continuing infection is suspected. Use an accurate thermometer placing it into the mouth for four minutes or as directed if it is an electronic thermometer.

The best time to take your temperature is first thing in the morning before getting out of bed. It should also be taken on at least one other occasion during the day particularly at a time when you have symptoms of fever or chill. Make sure that you have not had a hot or cold drink for some fifteen minutes before taking your temperature and that you follow the instructions on the thermometer carefully. Keep a record of the temperature readings over a two-week period. It is now considered that a temperature of up to 37.7°C (99.6°F) is normal. Usually the lowest values are in the morning and the peak values are in the late afternoon and early evening, with a variation of about 1°C (1.8°F) being quite normal. It is also normal to expect a very small temperature rise in women after they have ovulated in the middle of their menstrual cycle. Though your doctor may need to take your temperature in the course of his or her examination, your own temperature records may prove more useful.

TESTS

Over the last thirty years there has been an explosion in the number of laboratory tests that are now available for a wide variety of diseases. The difficulty for the doctor is to decide what tests should be performed now that the choice is so great. If you have been suffering with severe fatigue for a long time and it has been profound enough to disrupt your work or home life it is commonly accepted that a number of standard investigations should be carried out.

Urine tests

A simple urine test using a dipstick can test for protein, blood and sugar. This will detect kidney disease, kidney infection and diabetes.

Blood tests

There are several different blood tests that can be performed.

A full blood count This measures the haemoglobin (red blood pigment) level and looks at the number and types of red and white cells.

A low level of haemoglobin indicates anaemia, which has a number of causes. Changes in the size and shape of the blood cells may suggest iron deficiency or lack of vitamins B12 or folic acid and further blood tests may need to be performed to assess this properly.

White blood cells These are also measured in the blood count test. An increase in their number suggests that there is active infection or inflammation. There may be a shift in the balance of lymphocytes and neutrophils – the two major types of white cells – and this may again indicate an active infection or a recovery from a past infection. An increase in the number of eosinophils (another type of white cell) may suggest an allergy or parasitic infection and a low level of white blood cells may occur in certain blood disorders and diseases affecting the immune system.

ESR – erythrocyte sedimentation rate This is an old and well-established test that measures how quickly the red cells settle when placed in a vertical tube. A high ESR is usually caused by certain proteins in the blood which are formed in response to inflammation or infection. It does not tell us what the disease is, it just tells us that there is something going on. It is a cheap and fairly sensitive test, which usually suggests further tests to look for possible infection, arthritis, blood disorders and occasionally malignancy.

Serum electrolytes This involves measuring sodium, potassium and sometimes chloride. Low levels of sodium and potassium may occasionally be found in patients with fatigue and usually indicate a hormonal disturbance. High levels of potassium can occur in kidney failure.

Serum calcium This is often included routinely. An altered level may indicate a variety of ills that can show up because of fatigue, including hormonal and metabolic problems. If the calcium level is low or high the test usually needs to be repeated and the sample taken after you have fasted for several hours. Often sodium, potassium, calcium, protein, cholesterol and other tests are performed as a standard biochemical screen.

Kidney tests

These include measuring the blood levels of urea, creatinine or blood urea nitrogen. These are waste products of the metabolism that are excreted by the kidneys. A high level can indicate either kidney damage or, if there is acute illness, the rapid breakdown of tissues, especially muscles.

Liver function tests

These are a group of tests that include measurement of bilirubin – the pigment that when levels are too high causes jaundice – and the measurement of several liver enzymes. Increased levels of any one kind of several liver enzymes strongly suggest some kind of damage to the liver. The commonest cause is probably alcohol, but minor damage following viral infections that will fully recover is also an important and not infrequent cause.

Most liver diseases begin with slight increases in the blood levels of liver enzymes as they leak out from the damaged liver cells. Though rare it should be considered in patients with chronic fatigue who have minor blood liver abnormalities. In patients whose liver tests are abnormal it is customary to repeat these types of tests every month or two with the advice to stop drinking alcohol in the interim. Those patients whose results do not return to normal should be investigated further.

Thyroid function tests

Many doctors include some form of thyroid function test as routine in their assessment of a patient who has chronic fatigue. This is certainly a wise precaution in older patients and those with a family history of thyroid problems. Increased levels of thyroid hormones – T4 (thyroxine) or T3 (triiodothyronine) – are indeed indicative of an over-active thyroid. Low levels together with an increased level of thyroid stimulating hormone (TSH) suggest an under-active thyroid. There is considerable variation in the normal population and many people tolerate mild highs and lows without experiencing much ill-health.

Nutritional investigations

The tests described so far may have already assessed the imbalances of the minerals sodium, potassium and iron, vitamin B12 or folic acid. Other tests may need to be carried out if your doctor suspects that nutritional deficiency is a possible cause of your fatigue.

Serum ferritin   This is an extremely sensitive test for iron deficiency and is more specific than just measuring the level of haemoglobin. It will detect slight iron deficiency – a potential cause of mild fatigue – and should be considered in anyone with a low or borderline haemoglobin of between 11 and 12.5 grams per decilitre. Menstruating women and some vegetarians may be particularly at risk of mild iron deficiency. Measuring serum iron and total iron binding capacity (TIBC) is a useful alternative when serum ferritin is not available.

Serum vitamin B12 and serum and/or red cell folate These can also be measured by most hospital laboratories. They should be performed if the clinical picture suggests you have a deficiency or if the full blood count shows enlarged red cells (macrocytosis). Occasionally high levels occur in patients with liver disease or in those taking large amounts of vitamin B supplements and sometimes in people with bowel disorders where there is excess production of these vitamins in the gut which have then been absorbed into the bloodstream.

Other B vitamins Specialised tests to measure vitamin B1 (thiamin), vitamin B2 (riboflavin), vitamin B3 (nicotinamide) and vitamin B6 (pyridoxine) can be performed at certain laboratories. Though rarely performed they should be given some consideration especially to people who have fatigue together with depression and anxiety and other possible features of deficiency. Many of these vitamins are measured by assessment of the activity of an enzyme in the blood that requires the particular vitamin to work. A reduced level of activity of this enzyme is highly suggestive of deficiency.

Red cell magnesium Some but not all researchers have recorded low levels of red cell magnesium but normal serum magnesium in patients with chronic fatigue. A low level suggests that it might be worth trying a course of magnesium supplementation as tablets or by injection. The test should be easily performed by most good laboratories. Women with premenstrual syndrome seem to be particularly prone to have a low red cell magnesium level.

Other nutritional tests   Many other vitamins and minerals can be measured but this will only occasionally be useful. The role that other nutrients play in chronic fatigue is probably very small unless there is a reduced resistance to infection. Certainly lack of the trace element zinc can be important and the elderly, alcoholics and those with a poor diet are at risk of deficiency. A serum zinc test taken when the patient has not eaten for four hours is the simplest way to check.

Tests for hidden infection

These should be considered if there is a continuing fever or other features suggest infection. There are many blood tests which assess the level of antibodies against specific types of infection. If a recent viral infection is suspected then a repeat sample taken ten to fourteen days later may show a change in blood tests which shows that the body is mounting a response to a specific type of infection. Occasionally it is useful to have samples analysed to see if there is a particular organism present, and tests on urine, stool, blood and throat or other swabs can be taken for this.

Sometimes a useful test is to measure the levels of immunoglobulins. These are proteins that are composed of a number of unspecified antibodies. Levels of immunoglobulins G, A and M can easily be measured. Occasionally low levels, especially of immunoglobulin A, may be discovered and this together with other abnormalities can predispose the patient to repeated chest, throat, ear or gastro-intestinal infections. High levels of immunoglobulin M is very suggestive of recent viral or other infection. Unfortunately it does not tell us what the infection is or whether it requires any specific treatment itself. Increased levels of immunoglobulins A and G may also indicate infection or a variety of conditions including rheumatoid arthritis, chronic inflammation, liver or kidney disease.

Muscle tests

These rarely need to be performed but should be considered in patients with marked muscle problems especially muscle weakness and pain. The muscle enzyme creatine kinase can be measured in the blood, and high levels indicate muscle inflammation or degeneration. There are a variety of other similar tests. Lactic acid, which accumulates in muscles during exercise, can also be measured in the blood. High levels have been reported in occasional patients with chronic fatigue syndrome and an elevated level in the blood may suggest a disturbance in muscle metabolism, deficiency of vitamin B1 (thiamin) or a more serious disorder of muscle metabolism. Occasionally it is useful to measure the level of lactic acid after exercise to see how quickly it falls. This may give some indication of the degree of disturbance in muscle metabolism. The advantage of these tests is that they are relatively easy to perform compared with other more detailed tests of muscle metabolism. Those tests and the tests that measure the electrical activity of muscles are usually performed by a neurologist in specialised centres.

X-ray

The X-ray most routinely performed is a chest X-ray and this should be done if there is a shortness of breath, cough or heart problems.

ECG/EKG

This test to measure the electrical activity of the heart again should be done only if there are palpitations, high blood pressure or other indications of heart disease.

Other tests

There are numerous other tests, many of which are quite specialised, assessing hormonal function, disturbances in metabolism, tests for different types of arthritis and tests for rare conditions where the immune system produces anti-bodies against healthy tissues – auto-immune diseases. Specific tests which look further at kidney function, liver function and tests of absorption and digestion again sometimes need to be performed but almost only if one or more of the above tests are abnormal.

Interpretation of results

There is usually no difficulty determining what the results mean if they are either very normal or abnormal. The difficulty arises if there are only mild abnormalities which is not an uncommon situation. It then becomes particularly important to consider the whole picture of the patient's illness: the symptoms, findings from the examination and other details. Occasionally minor abnormalities can be ignored but usually a safe policy is to repeat the test either immediately or after several weeks have elapsed. When nutritional investigations show a borderline level of a nutrient, especially one of the lesser B vitamins or iron, it is perfectly justifiable to give a course of these for two or three months and if necessary repeat the test again.

It should always be remembered that it is bad medicine simply to treat a piece of paper and priority should be given to understanding the patient's problems and responding to them rather than the test result in isolation.

SUMMARY OF SURVEYS OF PATIENTS WITH CHRONIC FATIGUE

Main author	Subjects	Assessment	Findings
Morrison 1980	176 Subjects 123 Women 53 Men	Case records assessed retrospectively	39% Physically ill 41% Mentally ill 12% Physically and mentally ill
Marrie et al 1987	73 Subjects with post-viral illness	Laboratory investigations	Many with evidence of recent E-B viral 18% With abnormal liver function tests
Buchwald et al 1987	21% of 500 clinic attendees were fatigued	By interview	40 of those with CFS had E-B viral 78% Depressed mood changes 60% Anxious
Kroenke et al 1988	24% of 1159 patients with fatigue 102 of 276 with CFS assessed further	Interview and examination Interview, examination and laboratory investigations	6% Physically ill 1% Mentally ill on initial assessment 3% Hidden infection 9% Elevated ESR 12% Other minor blood abnormalities
Manu et al 1988	141 subjects with chronic fatigue	Physical and psychological assessments	5% Physically ill

Valdini et al 1988	45% of 254 clinic attendees with fatigue	Interview and case note inspection	27% Diagnosed as depressed, anxious or stressed
Valdini et al 1989	22 Subjects with CFS	Interview, examination and tests	5% Active infection 5% Past infection 5% Alcohol excess 18% Possible drug side-effects
Lloyd et al 1990	42 Subjects with post-infective syndrome	Interview and investigations	None with undiagnosed physical illness Some with minor immune changes
Kirk et al 1990	154 Subjects with chronic fatigue	Interview and case note inspection	37% With primarily psychological problems – anxiety and depression
Sharpe et al 1992	177 Adults with CFS	Interview, examination and tests	3% Elevated ESR 4% White cell changes 3–7% Minor liver test abnormalities 1% Elevated creatinine kinase No new major illnesses diagnosed

REFERENCES

1. Morrison, J.D., 'Fatigue as a present complaint in family practice', *Journal of Family Practitioners*, 1980; 10: 795–801.
2. Marrie, T.J., Ross, L., Montague, T.J., Doan, B., 'Post-viral fatigue syndrome', *Clinical Ecology*, 1987; 5: 5–10.
3. Buchwald, D., Sullivan, J.L., Komaroff, A.L., 'Frequency of chronic active Epstein-Barr virus infection in a general medical practice', *JAMA*, 1987; 257: 2303–2307.
4. Manu, P., Lane, T.J., Matthews, D.A., 'The frequency of chronic fatigue syndrome in patients with persistent fatigue,' *Annals Int. Med.*, 1988; 109: 554–556.

5. Kroenke, K., Wood, D.R., Mangelsdorff, B., Meier, N.J., Powell, J.D., 'Chronic fatigue in primary care', *JAMA*, 1988; 260: 929–934.

6. Valdini, A., Steinhardt, S., Valicenti, J., Jaffe, A., 'A one year follow up of fatigued patients', *Jour. Fam. Prac.* 1988; 26: 33–38.

7. Valdini, A., Steinhardt, S., Feldman, E., 'The usefulness of a standard battery of laboratory tests in investigating chronic fatigue in adults', *Fam. Pract.*, 1989; 6: 286–291.

8. Lloyd, A.R., Hickie, I., Boughton, C.R., Spencer, O., Wakefield, D., 'Prevalence of chronic fatigue syndrome in an Australian population', *Med. Jour. Australia*, 1990; 153: 522–528.

9. Kirk, J. et al., 'Chief complaint of fatigue: a prospective study', *Journal of Family Practice*, 1990; 30: 33–9.

10. Sharpe, M., Horton, K., Seagroatt, B., Pasvol, G. 'Follow-up patients presenting with fatigue to an infectious diseases clinic'. BMJ. 1992; 305: 147–152.

CONCLUSION

Undoubtedly, the onus is upon the doctor and support staff to take patients' complaints seriously, particularly when fatigue is severe enough to disrupt work or home life. The presence of other physical symptoms, including but not confined to fever, weight loss, muscle and joint pains, are more indicative of physical disorder than psychological or mood problems.

Most of the tests necessary to assess those with chronic fatigue state properly can be performed by a district hospital laboratory, though occasionally some tests have to be sent to specialised centres.

Careful physical assessment is an essential part of treating chronic fatigue states, either because *physical* cause may be found or, having been excluded, there is a considerable degree of reassurance for both the patient and the physician. Diligence, however, is the keynote to detecting physical problems in those with persistent fatigue states.

Glossary

Chronic E-B virus syndrome This term was favoured in the mid-1980s by the Americans who described a clinical picture identical to that of ME, but in association with sore throat and repeated or chronic swollen, painful neck glands. Very often such patients on blood testing had evidence of recent or continuing infection with the glandular fever virus.

Chronic fatigue syndrome The term chronic fatigue syndrome is the one preferred by many doctors, particularly in the United States, and by myself. It is non-committal and simply descriptive. This is the term that I have used throughout most of the book, though occasionally it has been appropriate to use the term myalgic encephalomyelitis (ME), post-viral, or post-infective fatigue syndromes.

It is probably best to consider chronic fatigue syndrome as the all-encompassing term. Within this term there are groups of those with post-infective fatigue, many of whom will be due to a viral infection, and some of these sufferers would qualify correctly for the term ME. There are, however, many other physical and psychological factors contributing to fatigue. Because I have attempted to cover most of this territory in the book, it is more appropriate to use the term chronic fatigue syndrome than any other.

Depression Reduction in mood. This is simply a descriptive term used to indicate feelings of unhappiness. They can be mild or severe. Depression can occur as a result of a physical illness, changes in body and brain chemistry, or as a reaction to stressful life situations. Depression is a common feature of chronic fatigue syndrome and its presence should not be interpreted as meaning that there is no physical component to the illness.

Fatigue Weariness from labour of body or mind. This could be either physical or mental.

Fibromyalgia Literally painful and tender muscles. This occurs not infrequently in patients with chronic fatigue syndrome, but is a condition in its own right to which there are both physical and psychological components.

Myalgic encephalomyelitis (ME) A syndrome of chronic fatigue accompanied by other symptoms. This usually includes abnormal muscle fatigue on exercise, poor memory or concentration and painful muscles. It well describes a clinical picture which often follows on from a viral infection, such as the glandular fever virus or several viruses that cause gastro-enteritis. The use of the term is best confined to those with a particular pattern of nerve and muscle symptoms that have followed on from a viral infection.

Post-infective fatigue syndrome Again, a more general term for fatigue following any type of infection, viral, bacterial, parasitic or fungal.

Post-viral fatigue syndrome Fatigue following any virus infection, which could include the glandular fever (Epstein-Barr) virus, or any other virus that typically causes a sore throat, gastro-enteritis or other infection.

Stamina Staying power. This is often reduced in patients with chronic fatigue syndrome in contrast to strength.

Strength The quality of being strong. This is rarely reduced in those with chronic fatigue or ME in contrast to stamina.

Acknowledgements

This book could not have been written without the invaluable contributions of many to whom recognition is due. Most important are the many doctors and other scientists whose work has resulted in numerous publications on the subject of fatigue. Many of their names are included in the text, and details of the relevant publications are included in the References section which follows. Their work deserves wider appreciation and I and many of my own patients have cause to be grateful to them.

Several of my colleagues deserve special mention: Dr Stephen Davies, Dr John Howard, Mr Adrian Hunnisett and staff at Biolab Medical Unit in London; my own secretarial staff, Judy Watts and Ann English; the staff of the Sussex Postgraduate Medical Centre, Brighton; those at The Hale Clinic in London, and Michelle Apsey from the Women's Nutritional Advisory Service. In the section on Complementary Therapies I was greatly helped by Julian Barker, medical herbalist, Deryn Bell, osteopath and Paul Lundberg, acupuncturist to whom thanks are due.

Particular thanks is due to my wife Maryon whose support and encouragement were essential to the production of the book. She also helped write much of the dietary sections of Part II. I am also grateful to Lavinia Trevor of the William Morris Agency for her steady guiding hand from the book's inception to its completion.

Final thanks goes to Jayne Booth, who had the unenviable task of editing the initial manuscript into the finished text.

Responsibility for any errors, that may have escaped my attention, rests with myself.

I hope too that many readers, public and professionals alike, will have cause to be grateful to those who have assisted with this book's production.

References

CHAPTER 1 – REFERENCES

1. Jenkins, R. and Mowbray, W. (eds), *Post-Viral Fatigue Syndrome*, John Wiley & Sons, Chichester, UK, 1990.
2. Behan, P., Goldberg, G. and Mowbray, J.F., 'Post-viral fatigue syndrome', *British Medical Bulletin* 47 No. 4, 1991.
3. Kendell, R.E., 'Chronic fatigue, viruses and depression', *The Lancet*, 1991; 337: 160–162.
4. Kennedy, H.G., 'Fatigue and fatigability', *British Journal of Psychiatry*, 1988; 153: 1–5.

MEDICAL REFERENCES

1. Morrison, J.D., 'Fatigue as a present complaint in family practice', *Journal of Family Practitioners* 1980; 10: 795–801.
2. Gold, M.S., Pottash, A.L.C. and Extein, I., 'Hypothyroidism in depression', *Journal of the American Medical Association*, 1981; 245: 1919–1922.
3. Marrie, T.J., Ross, L., Montague, T.J. and Doan, B., 'Post-viral fatigue syndrome', *Clinical Ecology*, 1987; 5: 5–10.
4. Manu, P., Lane, T.J. and Matthews, D.A., 'The frequency of chronic fatigue syndrome in patients with persistent fatigue', *Annals International Medicine*, 1988; 109: 554–556.
5. Kroenke, K., Wood, D.R., Mangelsdorff, B., Meier, N.J. and Powell, J.D., 'Chronic fatigue in primary care', *JAMA*, 1988; 260: 929–934.
6. Valdini, A., Steinhardt, S. and Feldman, E., 'The usefulness of a

standard battery of laboratory tests in investigating chronic fatigue in adults', *Family Practitioner*, 1989; 6: 286–291.

7. Lloyd, A.R., Hickie, I., Boughton, C.R., Spencer, O. and Wakefield, D., 'Prevalence of chronic fatigue syndrome in an Australian population', *Medical Journal of Australia*, 1990; 153: 522–528.

8. Wood, G.C., Bentall, R.P., Gopfert, N. and Edwards, R.H.T., 'The comparative psychiatric assessment of patients with chronic fatigue syndrome and muscle disease', *Psychological Medicine*, 1991; 21: 619–628.

9. Sharpe, M., Horton, K., Seagroatt, B. and Pasvol, G., 'Follow-up patients presenting with fatigue to an infectious disease clinic', *British Medical Journal*, 1992; 305: 147–152.

CHAPTER 2 – REFERENCES

1. David, A.S., Wessely, S. and Pelosi, A.J., 'Post viral fatigue syndrome: time for a new approach', *British Medical Journal*, 1988; 296: 696–699.

2. Wessely, S. (editorial), 'Chronic fatigue syndrome', *Journal of Neurology, Neurosurgery, Psychiatry*, 1991; 54: 669–671.

3. Wessely, S. and Powell, R., 'Fatigue syndromes: a comparison of chronic "post-viral" fatigue with neuromuscular and effective disorder', *Journal of Neurology, Neurosurgery, Psychiatry*, 1989; 52: 940–948.

4. Hickie, I., Lloyd, A., Wakefield, D. and Parker, G., 'The psychiatric status of patients with the chronic fatigue syndrome', *British Journal Psychiatry*, 1990; 156: 534–540.

5. Kruesi, M.J.P., Dale, J. and Straus, S.E., 'Psychiatric diagnoses in patients with chronic fatigue syndrome', *Journal of Clinical Psychology*, 1989; 50: 53–56.

6. Ray, Colette, 'Interpreting the role of depression in chronic fatigue syndrome', Jenkins, R. and Mowbray, J. (eds), in *Post-Viral Fatigue Syndrome*, John Wiley & Sons, Chichester, UK, 1991 (pp. 93–113).

7. Hall, R.C.W., *et al.*, 'Physical illness manifesting as psychiatric disease', *Archives of General Psychiatry*, 1980; 37: 989–995.

8. Koranyi, E.K., 'Morbidity and rate of undiagnosed physical illness in a psychiatric clinic population', *Archives of General Psychiatry*, 1979; 36: 414–419.

9. Gold, M.S., Pottash, A.L.C. and Extein, I., 'Hypothyroidism in depression', *Journal of the American Medical Association* 1981; 245: 1919–1922.

10. Bannister, P., Mortimer, A., Shapiro, L. and Simms, A.C.P., 'Thyroid function screening of psychiatric in-patient admissions: a worthwhile procedure?', *Journal of the Royal Society Medicine*, 1987; 80: 77–78.

11. Cadie, M., Nye, F.J. and Storey, P. 'Anxiety and depression after infectious mononucleosis', *British Journal of Psychiatry*, 1976; 128: 559–61.

12. White, T.D., 'Psychological and physical factors in post-infectious fatigue syndromes', presented at: Symposium on Psychological Management of Fatigue Syndromes, London, 20 September 1991.

CHAPTER 3 – REFERENCES

1. Mowbray, J., 'Enteroviruses and Epstein-Barr virus in ME', in Jenkins, R. and Mowbray, J.F. (eds), *Post-Viral Fatigue Syndrome*, John Wiley & Sons, Chichester, UK, 1991 (pp. 61–74).

2. Jones, J.F., *et al.*, 'Evidence of Epstein-Barr virus infection in patients with persistent unexplained illnesses: elevated anti-early antigen antibodies', *Annals of Internal Medicine*, 1985; 102: 1–7.

3. Hamblin, T.J., 'Immunological reasons for chronic ill health after infectious mononucleosis', *British Medical Journal*, 1983; 287: 85–88.

4. Buchwald, D., *et al.*, 'A chronic illness characterised by fatigue and neurologic disorders, and active human herpes virus type 6 infection', *Annals of Internal Medicine*, 1992; 116: 103–112.

5. Editorial, 'Epstein-Barr virus Silver Anniversary', *The Lancet*, 1989; 1: 1171–1173.

6. Borysiewicz, L.K., *et al.*, 'Epstein-Barr virus – specific immune defects in patients with persistent symptoms following infectious mononucleosis', *Quarterly Journal of Medicine*, 1986; 226: 111–121.

7. Editorial, 'EBV and persistent malaise', *The Lancet*, 1985; 1: 1017–1018.

8. Peters, T.J. and Preedy, V.R., 'Pathological changes in skeletal muscles in ME: implications for management', in Jenkins, R. and Mowbray, J., (eds) *Post-Viral Fatigue Syndrome*, John Wiley &

Sons, Chichester, UK, 1991, (pp. 137–146).

9. Bowles, N.E. and Archard, L.C., 'Persistent virus infection of muscle in patients with post-viral fatigue syndrome', in Jenkins, R. and Mowbray, J., (eds) *Post-Viral Fatigue Syndrome*, John Wiley & Sons, Chichester, UK, 1991, (pp. 147–166).

10. Gow, J.W., *et al.*, 'Enteroviral RNA sequences detected by polymerase chain reactions in muscles of patients with post-viral fatigue syndrome', *British Medical Journal*, 1991; 302: 692–696.

11. Archard, L.C., *et al.*, 'Post-viral fatigue syndrome: the persistence of enteroviral RNA in muscle and elevated creatine kinase', *Journal of the Royal Society of Medicine*, 1988; 81: 326–329.

12. Marrie, T.J., Ross, L., Montague, T.J. and Doan, B., 'Post-viral fatigue syndrome', *Clinical Ecology*, 1987; 5: 5–10.

13. Riley, M.S., *et al.*, 'Aerobic work capacity in patients with chronic fatigue syndrome', *British Medical Journal*, 1990; 301: 953–956.

14. Arnold, D.L., Bore, P.J., Radda, G.K., Stiles, P. and Taylor, D.J., 'Excessive intracellular acidosis of skeletal muscle on exercise in a patient with post-viral exhaustion/fatigue syndrome', *The Lancet*, 1984; 1: 1367–1369.

15. Pacy, P.J., Read, M., Peters, T.J. and Halliday, D., 'Post-absorptive whole body leucine kinetics and quadrecepts muscle protein synthetic rate (MPSR) in the post-viral syndrome', *Clinical Science*, 1988; 75: 36–37.

16. Behan, P.O., Behan, W.M.H. and Bell, E.J., 'Post-viral fatigue syndrome – an analysis of the findings in fifty cases', *Journal of Infection*, 1985; 10: 211–222.

17. Landay, A.L., Jessop, C., Lennette, E.T. and Levy, J.A., 'Chronic fatigue syndrome: clinical condition associated with immune activation', *The Lancet*, 1991; 2: 707–712.

18. Yousef, G., *et al.*, 'Chronic enterovirus infection in patients with post-viral fatigue syndrome', *The Lancet*, 1988; 1: 146–150.

19. Halpin, D. and Wessely, S., 'VP-1 antigen in chronic post-viral fatigue syndrome', *The Lancet*, 1989; 1: 1028–1029.

20. Komaroff, A.L., Geiger, A.M. and Wormsely, S., 'IgG subclass deficiencies in chronic fatigue syndrome', *The Lancet*, 1988; 1: 1288–1289.

21. MacWilliam, K., Dadswell, J.V. and Tillett, H., 'Antiviral titres, lymphocyte reactions and low IgA levels in patients with recurrent or persistent symptoms', *The Lancet*, 1985; 1: 764–765.

CHAPTER 4 – REFERENCES

1. Holmes, G.P., *et al.*, 'Chronic fatigue syndrome: A working case definition', *Annals of Internal Medicine*, 1988; 108: 387–389.
2. Weatherall, D.J., Ledingham, J.G.G. and Warrell, D.A. (eds), *Oxford Textbook of Medicine*, section 5, 'Infections'.
3. Mackowiak, P.A., Wasserman, S.S. and Levine, M.M., 'A critical appraisal of 98.6°F, the upper limit of the normal body temperature, and other legacies of Carl Reinhold August Wimberlich', *Journal of the American Medical Association*, 1992; 268: 1578–1580.
4. Weir, W.R.C., 'The presentation, investigation and diagnosis of patients with post-viral fatigue syndrome in an infectious diseases clinic', in Jenkins, R. and Mowbray, J. (eds), *Post-Viral Fatigue Syndrome*, John Wiley & Sons, Chichester, UK, 1991 (pp. 247–54).
5. Galland, L., 'The effect of intestinal microbes on systemic immunity', in Jenkins, R. and Mowbray, J. (eds), *Post-Viral Fatigue Syndrome*, John Wiley & Sons, Chichester, UK, 1991 (pp. 405–430).

CHAPTER 5 – REFERENCES

1. Behan, P.O., 'Diagnostic and clinical guidelines for doctors', (booklet published by the ME Association, Stanhope House, High Street, Stanford-le-Hope, Essex SS17 0HA).
2. Holmes, G.P., *et al.*, 'Chronic fatigue syndrome: a working case definition', *Annals of Internal Medicine*, 1988; 108: 387–389.
3. Weatherall, D.G., Ledingham, J.G.G. and Warrell, D.A. (eds), *Oxford Textbook of Medicine*, 1st edition 1984.

CHAPTER 6 – REFERENCES

1. Goodhart, R.S. and Shils, M.E., *Modern Nutrition in Health and Disease*, 6th edition, Lea & Feabiger, Philadelphia, USA, 1980.
2. Alpers, D.H., Clouse, R.E. and Stenson, W.F., *Manual of Nutritional Therapeutics*, 2nd edition, Little, Brown & Company, Boston, USA, 1988.

3. Passmore, R. and Eastwood, M.A., *Human Nutrition and Dietetics*, Churchill Livingstone, Edinburgh, 1986.
4. Davies, S. and Stewart, A., *Nutritional Medicine*, Pan Books, London, 1987.

CHAPTER 7 – REFERENCES

1. Lange, J., 'Concerning the disease of the virgins', in Ralph H. Major, *Classic Descriptions of Disease*. 3rd edition, Charles C. Thomas, Springfield, USA (pp. 487–489).
2. Gregory, J., Foster, K., Tyler, H. and Wiseman, M., *The Dietary and Nutritional Survey of Adults*, HMSO, London, 1990.
3. Department of Health, *Report on Health and Social Subjects 41: Dietary reference values for food, energy and nutrients for the United Kingdom*, HMSO, London, 1991.
4. Beutler, E., Larsh, S.E. and Gurney, C.W., 'Iron therapy in chronically fatigued non-anaemic women: a double-blind study', *Annals of Internal Medicine*, 1960; 52: 378–390.
5. Bull, N. and Barber, S., 'Food habits of 15–25 year olds: Dietary patterns and nutrient intakes of young women', *Health Visitor*, 1984; 57: 84–86.
6. Wood, M.M. and Elwood, P.C., 'Symptoms of iron deficiency anaemia. A community survey', *British Journal of Preventative and Social Medicine*, 1966; 20: 117–121.
7. Editorial, *The Lancet*, 1968; vol 1: 462–463.
8. Editorial, 'Happiness is: Iron', *British Medical Journal*, 1986; 292: 969–970.
9. Valberg, L.S., Sorbie, J., Ludwig, J. and Pelletier, O., 'Serum ferritin in the iron status of Canadians', *Canadian Medical Association Journal*, 1976; 114: 417–421.
10. Cook, J.D., Skikne, B.S., Lynch, S.R. and Reusser, N.E., 'Estimates of iron deficiency in the US population', *Blood*, 1986; 68: 726–731.
11. Wilson, J.F., Lahey, N.E. and Heiner, D.C., 'Studies of iron metabolism', *Journal of Paediatrics*, 1974; 84: 335–344.
12. Oski, F.A., 'Iron deficiency – facts and fallacies', *Paediatric Clinics of North America*, 1985; 32: 493–497.
13. Aukett, M.A., Parks, Y.A., Scott, P.H. and Wharton, B.A., 'Treatment with iron increases, weight gain and psychomotive

development', *Archives of Diseases in Childhood*, 1986; 61: 849–857.

CHAPTER 8 – REFERENCES

1. Cox, I.M., Campbell, M.J. and Dowsom, D., 'Red blood cell magnesium and chronic fatigue syndrome', *The Lancet*, 1991; 337: 757–760.
2. Cadell, J.L., Saier, F.L. and Thomason, C.A., 'Parental magnesium load tests in post-partum American women', *American Journal of Nutrition*, 1975; 28: 1099–1104.
3. Spatling, L. and Spatling, G., 'Magnesium supplementation in pregnancy. Double-blind study', *British Journal of Obstetrics and Gynaecology*, 1988; 95: 120–125.
4. Lennon, E.G., Lemann, J., Piering, W.F. and Larsson, L.S., 'The effect of glucose upon urinary kation excretion during chronic extracellular volume expansion in normal man', *Journal of Clinical Investigation*, 1974; 53: 1424–1433.
5. Lindeman, R.D., *et al.*, 'The influence of various nutrients on urinary diphan and kation excretion', *Journal of Laboratory and Clinical Medicine*, 1967; 70: 236–245.
6. McCollister, R.J., 'Urinary excretion of magnesium in man following the ingestion of ethanol', *American Journal of Clinical Nutrition*, 1983; 12: 415–419.
7. van Dokkum, W., 'The effect of high-animal and high-vegetable protein on mineral balance and bowel function of young men', *British Journal of Nutrition*, 1986; 56: 341–348.
8. Stebbing, J., Chernow, M.O. and Franz, K.B., 'Reactive hypoglycaemia and magnesium', *Magnesium Bulletin*, 1982; 2: 131–134.
9. McNair, P., Christiansen, C. and Transbol, 'The effect of menopause and oestrogen substitution therapy on magnesium metabolism', *Mineral and Electrolyte Metabolism*, 1984; 10: 84–87.
10. Frizel, D., Coppen, A. and Marks, V., 'Plasma magnesium and calcium in depression', *British Journal of Psychiatry*, 1969; 115: 1375–7.
11. Stendig-Lindberg, G. and Rudy, N., 'Predictors of maximum voluntary contraction force of Quadriceps Femoris Muscle in Man.' *Magnesium*, 1983; 2: 93–104.

12. Howard, J., 'Muscle action, trace elements and related nutrients: the myothermogram', in Chazot, G., Abdulla, M. and Arnaud, P. (eds), *Current Trends in Trace Elements Research: Proceedings of International Symposium on Trace Elements, Paris, 1987*, Smith-Gordon, London, 1989: 79–85.

13. Clague, J.E., Edwards, R.H.T. and Jackson, M.J., 'Intravenous magnesium loading in chronic fatigue syndrome', *The Lancet*, 1992; 2: 124–5.

14. Howard, J.Mc.L., Davies, S. and Hunnisett, A., 'Magnesium and chronic fatigue syndrome', *The Lancet*, 1992; 2: 426.

CHAPTER 9 – REFERENCES

1. Gregory, J., Foster, K., Tyler, H. and Wiseman, M., *The Dietary and Nutritional Survey of Adults*, London, HMSO, 1990.

2. Subar, A.F., Block, G. and James, L.D., 'Folate intake and food sources in the US population', *American Journal of Clinical Nutrition*, 1989; 50: 508–16.

3. Smidt, L.J., Cremin, F.M., Grivetti, L.E. and Clifford, A.J., 'The influence of folate status and polythenol intake on thiamine status of Irish women', *American Journal of Clinical Nutrition*, 1990; 52: 1077–8.

4. Morgan, A.G., *et al.*, 'A nutritional survey in the elderly: Haematological aspects', *International Journal of Vitamin and Nutrition Research*, 1973; 43: 461–471.

5. Morgan, A.G., *et al.*, 'A nutritional survey in the elderly: blood and urine vitamin levels', *International Journal of Vitamin and Nutrition Research*, 1975; 45: 448–460.

6. Goodwin, J.S., Goodwin, J.M. and Garry, P.J., 'The association between nutritional status and cognitive function in a healthy, elderly population', *Journal of the American Medical Association*, 1983; 249: 2917–2921.

7. Addis, G.M. and Bruncie, J., 'Water-soluble vitamin deficiency in the elderly', *Medical and Laboratory Sciences*, 1985; 42: 90–91.

8. Carney, M.W.P., Williams, D.G. and Sheffield, B.F., 'Thiamine and pyridoxine lack in newly-committed psychiatric patients', *British Journal of Psychiatry*, 1979; 135: 249–54.

9. Godfrey, P.S.A., *et al.*, 'The enhancement of recovery from psychiatric illness by methyl folate', *The Lancet*, 1990; 2: 392–395.

10. Vernon, D.I. and Stephen, J.M.L., 10th International Congress of Nutrition, Kyoto, 1975. Abstract 6340, p. 302.

11. Stewart, J.W., Harrison, W., Quitkin, F. and Baker, H., 'Low B6 levels in depressed out-patients', *Biological Psychiatry*, 1984; 19: 613–617.

12. Leevy, C., *et al.*, 'The incidence and significance of hypovitamin-aemia in a randomly selected municipal hospital population', *American Journal of Clinical Nutrition*, 1964; 17: 259–271.

13. Leevy, C., *et al.*, 'B complex vitamins in liver disease of the alcoholic', *American Journal of Clinical Nutrition*, 1965; 16: 339.

14. Ellis, F.R. and Nasser, S.A., 'Pilot study of vitamin B12 in the treatment of tiredness', *British Journal of Nutrition*, 1973; 30: 277–283.

15. Bell, I.R., *et al.*, 'Brief communication: vitamin B1, B2 and B6 augmentation of tricyclic antidepressant treatment in geriatric depression with cognitive dysfunction', *Journal of the American College of Nutrition*, 1992; 11: 159–163.

16. Jacobson, W., Wreghitt, T.G., Saich, T. and Nagington, J., 'Serum folate in viral and mycoplasmal infections', *Journal of Infection*, 1987; 14: 103–111.

CHAPTER 10 – REFERENCES

1. Goodhart, R.S. and Shils, M.E., *Modern Nutrition in Health and Disease*, 6th edition, Lea & Febiger, Philadelphia, USA, 1980.

2. Passmore, R. and Eastwood, M.A., *Human Nutrition and Dietetics*, 8th edition, Churchill Livingstone, Edinburgh, 1986.

3. Alpers, D.H., Clouse, R.E. and Stenson, W.F., *Manual of Nutritional Therapeutics*, Little, Brown & Co., Boston, USA, 1987.

4. Gershwin, N.E., Beech, R.S. and Hurley, L.S., *Nutrition and Immunity*, Academic Press Inc, Orlando, USA, 1985.

5. Lind, J., in R.H. Major, *Classic Descriptions of Disease*, 6th edition, Charles C. Thomas, Springfield, USA, 1965 (pp. 589–592).

6. Hodges, R.E., Baker, E.M., Hood, J., Sauberlich, H.E. and March, S.C., 'Experimental scurvy in man', *American Journal of Clinical Nutrition*, 1969; 22: 535–548.

7. Crandon, J.H., Mikal, S. and Landeau, B.R., 'Ascorbic acid deficiency in experimental and surgical subjects', *Proceedings of Nutrition Society*, 1953; 12: 273–279.

8. Hughes, R.E., 'Recommended daily amounts and biochemical roles – the vitamin C, carnitine, fatigue relationship', in Counsell, J.N. and Horning, D.H. (eds), *Vitamin C*, Applied Science Publishers, London, 1981.

9. Bruzina, R. and Suboticanec, K., 'Vitamin C and physical working capacity', in Hanck, A. and Hornig, D. (eds), *Vitamins – nutrients and therapeutic agents*, Hans Huber Publishers, Berne, 1985 (pp. 185–166).

10. Strydom, N.B., 'Heat intolerance, its detection and elimination in the mining industry', *South African Journal of Science*, 1980; 76: 154–156.

11. Friedland, J. and Paterson, D., 'Potassium and fatigue', *The Lancet*, 1988; 2: 961–962.

12. Whang, R., *et al.*, 'Hypomagnesaemia and hypokalaemia in 1000 treated ambulatory hypertensive patients', *Journal of the American College of Nutrition* 1982; 1: 317–322.

13. Dorup, I. and Clausen, T., 'The effects of potassium deficiency on growth and protein synthesis in skeletal muscle and hearts of rats', *British Journal of Nutrition*, 1989; 62: 269–284.

14. Ledbetter, M.L.S. and Lubin, M., 'The control of protein synthesis in human fibroblasts by intracellular potassium', *Experimental Cell Research*, 1977; 105: 223–236.

15. Zimran, A., Karaner, M., Plaskin, M. and Hershko, C., 'The incidence of hyperkalaemia induced by Indomethecin in a hospital population', *British Medical Journal*, 1985; 291: 107–108.

16. Haalboom, J.R.E., Deenstra, M. and Struyvenberg, A., 'Hypokalaemia induced by inhalation of Fenoterol', *The Lancet*, 1985; 1: 1125–1127.

17. Dyckner, T. and Wester, P-O., 'Magnesium treatment of diuretic induced hyponatremia with a preliminary report of a new aldosterone antagonist', *Journal of the American College of Nutrition*, 1982; 1: 149–153.

18. Swales, J.D., 'Salt substitutes and potassium intake', *British Medical Journal*, 1991; 303: 1084–1085.

19. Vanfraechem, J.H.P., *et al.*, *Biomedical and Clinical Aspects of Co-enzyme Q3*, Elsevier Science Publishers BV, 1981 (p. 235 et seq.).

CHAPTER 11 – REFERENCES

1. McCance, R.A., Luff, M.C. and Widdosson, E.E., 'Physical and emotional periodicity in women', *Journal of Hygiene*, 1937; 37: 571–612.
2. Ritchie, C.D. and Singkamani, R., 'Plasma pyridoxal-5′-phosphate in women with premenstrual syndrome', *Human Nutrition: Clinical Nutrition*, 1986; 46C: 75–80.
3. Abraham, G.E. and Lubran, M.M., 'Serum and red cell magnesium levels in patients with PMS', *American Journal of Clinical Nutrition*, 1981; 34: 2364–6.
4. Sherwood, R.A., Rocks, B.F., Stewart, A. and Saxton, R.S., 'Magnesium and the premenstrual syndrome', *Annals of Clinical Biochemistry*, 1986; 23: 667–670.
5. O'Brien, P.M.S., *Premenstrual Syndrome*, Blackwell Scientific Publications, Oxford, 1987.
6. Facchinetti, F., *et al.*, 'Oral magnesium successfully relieves premenstrual mood changes', *Obstetrics and Gynaecology*, 1981; 78: 177–181.
7. Chakmakjian, Z.H., Higgins, C.E. and Abraham, G.E., 'The effect of a nutritional supplement, Optivite for women, on premenstrual tension syndromes: effect of symptomatology, using a double-blind, cross-over design', *Journal of Applied Nutrition*, 1985; 37: 12.
8. Stewart, A., 'Assessment of nutritional deficiencies in women with premenstrual syndromes (PMS): clinical and biochemical effects of nutritional supplementation', *Journal of Reproductive Medicine*, 1987; 32: 435.
9. London, R.S., Bradley, L. and Chiamori, N.Y., 'Effect of nutritional supplement on premenstrual symptomatology in women with premenstrual syndrome: A double-blind longitudinal study', *Journal of the American College of Nutrition*, 1991; 10: 494–499.
10. Stewart, A., Tooley, S. and Stewart, M., 'The effect of a nutritional programme on premenstrual syndrome', *Journal of Complementary Medicine Research*, 1991; 5: 8–11.

CHAPTER 12 – REFERENCES

1. RCP Report, 'Food intolerance and food aversion', *Journal of the*

Royal College of Physicans, London, 1984: vol 8, number 2.

2. Brostoff, J. and Gamlin, L., *Food Allergy and Intolerance*, Bloomsbury, London, 1989.

3. Arnason, J.A., Gudjonsson, H., Freysdottir, J., Jonsdottir, I. and Valdimarsson, H., 'Do adults with high gliadin antibody concentrations have subclinical gluten intolerance?', *GUT*, 1992; 33: 194–7.

CHAPTER 13 – REFERENCES

1. Editorial, 'Yeast on skin', *British Medical Journal*, 1973; 2: 70.

2. Hay, R.J. and Mackenzie, D.W.R., 'Fungal infections (mycoses)', in Weatherall, D.J., Ledingham, J.G.G. and Warrell, D.N. (eds), *Oxford Textbook of Medicine*, Oxford University Press, Oxford, 1983; vol. 1; 5: 369–384.

3. James, J. and Warin, R.P., 'Assessment of the role of candida albicans and food yeasts in chronic urticaria', *British Journal of Dermatology*, 1971; 84: 227–230.

4. Sclafer, J., *L'Allergie à candida albicans*, Semaine Hopital, Paris, 1957; 33: 1330–1339.

5. Rufin, J.M. and Kayer, D., 'The effect of vitamin supplements on normal persons', *Journal of the American Medical Association*, 1944; 126: 823–825.

6. Holti, G., 'Candida allergy', in H.I. Winner and Rosalind Hurley (eds), *Symposium on Candida Infections*, Livingstone, Edinburgh, 1966 (p. 73).

7. Hurley, R., 'Inveterate vaginal thrush', *The Practitioner*, 1975; 215: 753–756.

8. Danna, P.L., Urban, C., Bellin, E. and Rahal, J., 'The role of candida in the pathogenesis of antibiotic-associated diarrhoea in elderly patients', *The Lancet*, 337; 1: 511–514.

9. Renfro, L., Feder, H.N., Lane, T.G., Manu, P. and Matthews, D.A., 'The yeast connection in 100 patients with chronic fatigue', *American Journal of Medicine*, 1989; 86: 165–168.

10. Dismukes, W.E., Scott Wade, J., Lee, J.Y., Dockery, B.K. and Hain, J.D., 'Randomised, double-blind trial of Nystatin therapy for the candidiasis hypersensitivity syndrome', *New England Journal of Medicine*, 1990; 323: 1717–1723.

11. Bennett, J.E., 'Searching for the yeast connection', *New England*

Journal of Medicine, 1990; 323: 1766–1767.
12. Wells, R.S., Higgs, J.N., MacDonald, A., Valdimarsson, H. and Holt, P.J.L., 'Familial chronic muco-cutaneous candidiasis', *Journal of Medical Genetics*, 1972; 9: 302–310.
13. 'Management of oral candidosis', *Drugs and Therapeutic Bulletin*, 1990; 28: 13–15.

CHAPTER 14 – REFERENCES

 1. Marks, V., 'Recognition and d6ifferential diagnosis of spontaneous hypoglycaemia', *Clinical Endocrinology*, 1992; 37: 309–316.
 2. Service, F.J., 'Hypoglycaemia and the post-prandial syndrome', *New England Journal of Medicine*, 1989; 321: 1472–1474.
 3. Rothstein, J.D., 'Endogenous benzodiazepene receptor ligands in idiopathic recurring stupor', *The Lancet*, 1992; 2: 1002–1004.
 4. McBride, S.J. and McCluskey, D.R., 'The treatment of chronic fatigue syndrome', *British Medical Bulletin*, 1991; 47: 895–907.
 5. Blau, J.N., 'Migraine: theories of pathogenesis', *The Lancet*, 1982; 1: 1202–1206.
 6. Lance, J.W., 'Treatment of migraine', *The Lancet*, 1992; 1: 1207–1209.
 7. Egger, W.J., Carter, C.M., Wilson, J., Turner, M.F. and Soothill, J.F., 'Is migraine food allergy?', *The Lancet*, 1983; 2: 865–869.
 8. Pelosi, A.J., *et al.*, 'A psychiatric study of idiopathic oedema', *The Lancet*, 1986; 2: 999–1002.
 9. MacGregor, G.A., *et al.*, 'Is "idiopathic" oedema idiopathic?', *The Lancet*, 1979; 1: 397–400.
10. Komaroff, A.L., 'Post-viral fatigue syndrome: a review of American research and practice', in Jenkins, R. and Mowbray, J. (eds), *Post-Viral Fatigue Syndrome*, John Wiley & Sons, Chichester, UK, 1991 (pp. 41–60).
11. Wysenbeek, A.J., *et al.*, 'Primary fibromyalgia and the chronic fatigue syndrome', *Rheumatology International*, 1991; 10: 227–229.
12. Banerji, N.K. and Hurwitz, L.J., 'Restless leg syndrome, with particular reference to its occurrence after gastric surgery', *British Medical Journal*, 1970; 4: 774–775.
13. Rodger, S.D., 'Possible relation between restless legs and anaemia in renal dialysis patients', *The Lancet*, 1991; 337: 1551.
14. Ekbom, K.A., 'Restless leg syndrome', *Neurology*, 1960; 10: 868–73.

15. von Scheele, C., 'Levodopa in restless legs', *The Lancet*, 1986; 2: 426–427.
16. Read, D.J., Feest, T.G. and Nassim, M.A., 'Clonazepam: effect of treatment for restless leg syndrome in uraemia', *British Medical Journal*, 1981; 383: 885–886.
17. Editorial, 'Snoring and sleepiness', *The Lancet*, 1985; 2: 925–926.
18. Rees, J., 'Snoring', *British Medical Journal*, 1981; 302: 860–861.
19. Partinen, M. and Palomaki, H., 'Snoring and cerebral infarction', *The Lancet*, 1985; 2: 1325–1326.
20. Heaton, K.W., *et al.*, 'Symptoms of irritable bowel syndrome in a British urban community: consulters and non-consulters', *Gastro-enterology*, 1992; 102: 1962–1967.
21. Drossman, D.A., *et al.*, 'Bowel patterns amongst subjects not seeking health care', *Gastroenterology*, 1982; 83: 592–594.
22. Whorwell, P.J., McCallum, M., Creed, F.H. and Roberts, C.T., 'Non-colonic features of irritable bowel syndrome', *Gut*, 1986; 27: 37–40.
23. Alun Jones, V., McLaughlan, P., Shorthouse, M., Workman, E. and Hunter, J.O., 'Food intolerance: a major factor in the pathogenesis of irritable bowel syndrome', *The Lancet*, 1982; 2: 1115–1117.
24. Whorwell, P.J., Prior, A. and Colgan, S.M., 'Hypnotherapy in severe irritable bowel syndrome: further experience', *Gut*, 1987; 28: 423–425.
25. Hunter, J.O., 'Food allergy – or enterometabolic disorder?', *The Lancet*, 1991; 2: 495–496.
26. Pilgrim, J.A., Standsfield, S. and Marmot, M., 'Low blood pressure, low mood?', *British Medical Journal*, 1992; 304: 75–78.
27. Mann, A., 'Psychiatric symptoms in low blood pressure', *British Medical Journal*, 1992; 304: 64–65.
28. Heseltine, D. and Potter, J.F., 'Post-prandial hypotension in elderly people', *Age and Ageing*, 1990; 19: 233–235.
29. Gershwin, M.E., Beech, R.S. and Hurley, L.S., *Nutrition and Immunity*, Academic Press Inc, Orlando, USA, 1985.

CHAPTER 15 – REFERENCES

1. Beaumont, G., 'Sleep disorders: their diagnosis and management in general practice', *Psychiatry in Practice*, 1992, Summer: 18–22.

Recommended reading

Below are a selection of books for lay readers on fatigue and some of the other topics covered in *Tired All The Time*.

Fatigue
Dr Anne Macintyre, *M.E. Post-Viral Fatigue Syndrome How to Live with It*, Thorsons, London, 1992.

Nutrition
Drs Stephen Davies and Alan Stewart, *Nutritional Medicine*, Pan Books, London, 1987.

McCance and Widdowson's *The Composition of Foods*, 4thedition, A.A. Paul and D.A.T. Southgate, HMSO, London, 1978.

Report on Health and Social Subjects 41. Dietary Reference Values for Food Energy and Nutrients for the United Kingdom. Report of the Panel on Dietary Reference Values of the Committee on Medical Aspects of Food Policy, HMSO, London, 1991.

Migraine
Dr John Mansfield, *The Migraine Revolution*, Thorsons, London, 1986.

Irritable bowel syndrome
Elizabeth Workman, Dr John Hunter and Dr Virginia Alun Jones, *The Allergy Diet*, Optima, London, 1988.

Premenstrual syndrome
Maryon Stewart, *Beat PMT Through Diet*, 2nd edition, Vermilion, 1992.

Useful addresses

The ME Association
Stanhope House, High Street, Stanford-Le-Hope, Essex SS17 0HA

ME Action
P.O. Box 1302, Wells, Somerset BA5 2WE
Tel: 0749 670799

Action Against Allergy
24–26 High Street, Hampton Hill, Middlesex TW12 1PD

British Society of Allergy and Environmental Medicine
34 Brighton Road, Banstead, Surrey SM17 1BS
Tel: 07373 61177

Women's Nutritional Advisory Service
P.O. Box 268, Lewes, East Sussex BN7 2QN
Tel: 0273 487366

British Homoeopathic Association
27a Devonshire Street, London W1N 1JJ
Tel: 071-935 2163

Samaritans
17 Uxbridge Road, Slough SL1 1SN
Tel: 0753 532713

Shiatsu Society
c/o 14 Oakdene Road, Redhill, Surrey RH1 6BT

British Acupuncture Register and Directory
34 Alderney Street, London SW1V 4UE
Tel: 071 8344 0112

Council for Acupuncture
Suite 1, 19A Cavendish Square, London W1M 9AD
Tel: 071 495 8153

The National Institute of Medical Herbalists
41 Hatherly Road, Winchester, Hants SO22 6RR
Tel: 0962 68776

The European School of Osteopathy
Littlejohn House, 1–4 Suffolk Street, London SW1 4HG
Tel: 0622 671 558

The Cranial Osteopathic Association
47B Baker Street, Enfield, Middx EN1 3QS
Tel: 081 367 5561

Index